2003

PCAT SUCCESS

TEST PREP

Dick R. Gourley, Pharm.D.
Greta A. Gourley, Pharm.D., Ph.D.

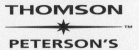
THOMSON
PETERSON'S

Australia • Canada • Mexico • Singapore • Spain • United Kingdom • United States

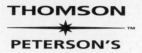

About The Thomson Corporation and Peterson's

With revenues of US$7.2 billion, The Thomson Corporation (www.thomson.com) is a leading global provider of integrated information solutions for business, education, and professional customers. Its Learning businesses and brands (www.thomsonlearning.com) serve the needs of individuals, learning institutions, and corporations with products and services for both traditional and distributed learning.

Peterson's, part of The Thomson Corporation, is one of the nation's most respected providers of lifelong learning online resources, software, reference guides, and books. The Education Supersite[sm] at www.petersons.com—the Internet's most heavily traveled education resource—has searchable databases and interactive tools for contacting U.S.-accredited institutions and programs. In addition, Peterson's serves more than 105 million education consumers annually.

For more information, contact Peterson's, 2000 Lenox Drive, Lawrenceville, NJ 08648; 800-338-3282; or find us on the World Wide Web at: www.petersons.com/about.

Sixth Edition

ISBN: 0-7689-1010-2

Printed in the United States of America

10 9 8 7 6 5 4 3 2 1   05 04 03

Contents

Introduction to Pharmacy Practice

HISTORICAL PERSPECTIVE

The origins of the profession of pharmacy can be traced back to ancient Babylonia-Assyria, Egypt, and Greece (approximately 3000 B.C.E.). Although very little is known of pharmacy at that time, fragments of knowledge remain. The word *pharmacy* and its derivatives can be traced this far back and to some degree explain the meaning of the Greek word *pharmakon*. Opinions are divided as to whether there were pharmacists in ancient Egypt, or rather, "physician assistants" who specialized in the preparation of pharmaceuticals.

Originally, pharmacy was the work of priests, but it later became part of the function of lay medical practitioners who combined both medicine and pharmacy. The birth of the European professional pharmacy was some time around 1240 when the German Emperor Frederick II issued "an edict that was to be the Magna Charta of the profession of pharmacy" (see Kramer and Urdang's *History of Pharmacy*, Lippincott, Philadelphia, 1963). As medicine and pharmacy grew and matured, the pharmacist became responsible for the preparation and dispensing of medications and in European societies became known as an apothecary. The physician became responsible for diagnosing and treating illness, while the pharmacist became responsible for the preparation and dispensing of medication. Thus, the dispensary.

Educationally, pharmacy has evolved from an apprenticeship that did not require any formal education to a sophisticated professional degree program. By 1900, pharmacy education was approximately 10 percent education and 90 percent practice. The first school of pharmacy in the United States was the Philadelphia School of Pharmacy and Sciences, founded in 1821. Early schools of pharmacy in the United States were privately owned and were used to educate physicians as well as pharmacists. The first state university to offer a program in pharmacy was the Medical College of South Carolina, founded in 1867.

The standard dictionary definition of pharmacy is "the art or practice of preparing, preserving, compounding, and dispensing drugs." However, the roles that the pharmacist has fulfilled have also included the following:

- Storing and purchasing medications
- Advising patients and other health-care providers on medications
- Manufacturing/Quality Control
- Pharmaceutical Sales
- Education
- Research

As technology advanced, the role of the pharmacist expanded in health care. In the 1960s, the clinical movement in pharmacy began, which led to pharmaceutical care.

PATIENT-CENTERED PHARMACEUTICAL CARE ERA

Since the 1960s, the pharmacy profession has moved toward a more patient-oriented rather than a product-oriented practice. This shift has come about from the increasing number of new drug products that have appeared on the market, with greater need for patient information about those drugs, as well as the increased cost of health care. Likewise, pharmacy education has moved from chemistry/laboratory-based education to biological/patient-care based. Automation has begun to replace the pharmacist as a dispenser of medications, and the need for patient education to resolve therapeutic dilemmas has been well documented. Thus, pharmacist responsibilities for patient education continue to expand.

Pharmaceutical care was first defined by R.L. Mikeal, et al, in 1975, as "the care that a given patient requires and receives which assures safe and rational drug usage." (Mikeal, R.L., R.P. Brown, H.L. Lazarus, and M.C Vinson. 1975. Quality of pharmaceutical care in hospitals. *Am. J. Hosp. Pharm.* 32:567-74.)

In 1980, D.C. Brodie suggested that pharmaceutical care include the determination of drug needs for a patient and the concept of a feedback mechanism to facilitate continuity of care. (Brodie, D.C., P.A. Parish, and J.W. Poston. 1980. Social needs for drugs and drug-related services. *Am. J. Pharm. Ed.* 51:369-85.)

C.D. Hepler described pharmaceutical care as "a covenantal relationship between a patient and a pharmacist in which the pharmacist performs drug-use–control functions (with appropriate knowledge and skill) governed by awareness of a commitment to the patient's interest." (Hepler, C. D. 1987. The third wave in pharmaceutical education and the clinical movement. *Am. J. Pharm. Ed.* 51:369-85.)

C.D. Hepler and L.M. Strand indicated that "pharmaceutical care is the responsible provision of drug therapy for the purpose of achieving a definite outcome that improves a patient's quality of life." (Hepler, C.D., and L.M. Strand. 1990. Opportunities and responsibilities in pharmaceutical care. *Am. J. Hosp. Pharm.* 47:533-43.)

J.A. Johnson and J.L. Bootman indicated that as a result of drug-related illnesses, ambulatory patients in the United States spend more than $76 billion annually. This sum exceeds the cost of drug therapy itself. The estimate does not include the indirect costs of drug-related illness, such as loss of work and productivity. (Johnson, J. A., and J.L. Bootman. 1995. Drug-related morbidity and mortality: a cost-of-illness model. *Arch. Intern. Med.* 155:1949-56.) Pharmacists are positioned to take a major role in improving patient compliance and to resolve this $76-billion problem. Managed care is demanding an increased level of pharmacist involvement in patient care to improve health care, as well as to control costs. Likewise, patients have become more aggressive in their quest for information about their medications and their diseases. Direct-to-consumer advertising has made an impact on the level of knowledge of the patient and heightened awareness of the need for information.

Patient-centered pharmaceutical care includes the following roles for the pharmacist:

1. **Patient Education**—discussing the correct way for the patient to take medication, educating the patient about his or her disease, and answering questions the patient has about the disease, drug therapy, or related matters. Health education is a necessity for the pharmacist.

2. **Monitoring**—the patient's medication therapy to assure that the drug is accomplishing its purpose and to assure that no side effects or adverse drug reactions are occurring, as well as to assess the patient's understanding of the disease and the drug therapy so as to improve patient compliance.

3. **Providing pharmacokinetic consultations**—providing information to physicians on drug absorption, drug excretion, and drug metabolism of specific drugs. This allows for individualized dosing that assures optimal drug therapy results.

4. **Relating drug information**—to physicians, nurses, dentists, and other health-care providers, as well as to the public.

5. **Prescribing**—pharmacists have traditionally had the responsibility of recommending over-the-counter drugs to patients. However, over the past several years, there have been changes in pharmacy practice laws in several states that provide for pharmacists prescribing under protocol and also for collaborative care agreements between pharmacists and physicians, as well as other health-care providers.

6. **Disease Management**—involves working with other health-care professionals to provide disease management for specific patient populations. For example, diabetes and asthma are two chronic diseases that pharmacists have been actively involved with as members of the disease management team.

Pharmacists are uniquely positioned to assume these roles as a consequence of their availability to the public, their education, and the trust that the public has in them. A Gallup Poll recognized pharmacists as the most trusted profession for the sixth year in a row. (McAneny, L. 1995. Annual honesty & ethics poll: racial divisions evident in rating of police, lawyers. *Gallup Poll News Service*. 126(3): 54.)

If you wish to read more about the pharmacist's responsibilities relating to patient-centered pharmaceutical care, we recommend the following references:

1. "Standards of Practice for the Profession of Pharmacy," *American Pharmacy* 19, no. 3 (1979): 31.

2. "Pharmacy in the 21st Century Conference: Executive Summary," *The Consultant Pharmacist* 5, no. 4 (April 1990): 226–233.

3. Manasse, Henri R., Jr. "Medication Use in an Imperfect World," *American Society of Hospital Pharmacists* 46 (1989): 929–44 and 1141–52.

4. Hepler, C.D. 1987. The third wave in pharmaceutical education: the clinical movement. *Am. J. Pharm. Ed.* 51: 369–384.

5. Cocolas, G.H. 1989. Pharmacy in the 21st-century conference: executive summary. *Am. J. Pharm. Ed.* Winter. 53(WS): 15–55.

6. Brodie, D.C., P.A. Parish, and J.W. Poston. 1987. Social needs for drugs and drug-related services. *Am. J. Pharm. Ed.* 51: 369–85.

7. Proceedings: Understanding and preventing drug misadventures. A multidisciplinary invitational conference sponsored by the ASHP Research and Education Foundation in cooperation with the American Medical Association, the American Nurses Association, and the American Society of Hospital Pharmacists. 1995. *Am. J. Health-Syst. Pharm.* 52: 369–416.

8. Gourley, D.R. 1989. Curriculum evolution: What progress have we made? *Am. J. Pharm. Ed.* 53: 375–9.

A 1975 study of the future of pharmacy practice and education, *Pharmacists for the Future*, provides an in-depth analysis of past and present trends in the pharmacy profession and discusses the roles that future pharmacists will fill. The following quotation is from the Millis Commission report, *Pharmacists for the Future*, the Report of the Study Commission on Pharmacy. Health Administration Press, Ann Arbor, 1975:

Pharmacy should be defined basically as a system which renders a health service by concerning itself with knowledge about drugs and their effects upon man and animal. Pharmacy generates knowledge about drugs, acquires relevant knowledge from the biological, chemical, physical, and behavioral sciences; it tests, organizes and applies that knowledge. Pharmacy translates a substantial portion of that knowledge into drug products and distributes them widely to those who require them. Pharmacy knowledge is disseminated to physicians, pharmacists, other health care providers and to the general public that drug knowledge and products may contribute to the health of individuals and to the welfare of society. The knowledge system of pharmacy through its therapeutic use is a substantial and significant segment of health care in the United States.

CAREER OPPORTUNITIES

Since the 1960s, pharmacy education and practice have undergone incredible changes. These changes continue to occur in the twenty-first century. Pharmacy is still evolving even though it is an old and honored profession. Job opportunities are available in a variety of areas, including, but not limited to, community pharmacy (independent practice or chain store), hospital pharmacy, the pharmaceutical industry, government, geriatric pharmacy services, and clinical practice in a variety of specialty areas such as nuclear pharmacy, pharmacotherapy, nutrition support practice, psychiatric practice, and oncology practice. Practice in managed care is still evolving, and in the future there will be practice opportunities in areas that have not yet been identified.

Educational opportunities beyond a pharmacy degree include graduate education in the pharmaceutical and medical sciences or in other health-care fields (medicine, dentistry, etc.). The opportunity to continue educationally in a collateral area, such as combining a pharmacy career with law or with an M.B.A., exists as well.

As you can easily see, job opportunities are varied. Individuals who complete either a Bachelor of Science in pharmacy (B.S.) or a Doctor of Pharmacy degree (Pharm.D.) have many opportunities available to them. Postgraduate education also offers an excellent opportunity for continuing one's education and building upon the basic pharmacy education.

The following are brief descriptions of some of the career opportunities available to individuals who complete the basic requirements for pharmacy licensure.

Note: The American Council on Pharmaceutical Education (ACPE) announced in July of 1997 that the Pharm.D. would be the only accredited entry-level degree in pharmacy. Even though some schools and colleges still offer a B.S., these programs will be phased out over the next five to eight years.

Community/Ambulatory Pharmacy

Community pharmacists are increasingly becoming practitioners who provide a variety of health-care services to patients, including medications, patient education on disease and drugs, immunizations, allergy shots, and therapeutic drug monitoring. In addition to having responsibility for the distribution of drugs to patients, the pharmacist is also responsible for educating the patient about medications.

Because of the ever-increasing quantity of pharmaceutical knowledge, professionals in other areas of health care are turning more frequently to pharmacists for advice and assistance. Pharmacists contribute information that will be helpful in selecting the best drug therapy for a patient and help physicians monitor the patient's progress. Pharmacists must detect possible adverse reactions patients may have to drugs and any interactions that may occur, including drug-drug, drug-food, and drug-disease interactions. They have an opportunity and responsibility to advise patients in their use of nonprescription drugs. In addition, they must make recommendations to patients and other health professionals for avoiding problems with drug use.

The practice of community pharmacy is also a business. In addition to their patient-care activities, pharmacists must also manage people, resources, and time. The opportunity for community involvement and the respect of the patient make community practice exciting. Opportunities are available in rural and metropolitan areas as well as in a variety of settings, such as apothecaries, chain stores, and independent community pharmacies.

For more information about community/ambulatory practice, contact the **American Pharmaceutical Association (APhA),** 2215 Constitution Ave. NW, Washington, DC 20037-2985; 202-628-4410; fax: 202-783-2351; www.aphanet.org.

Institutional Pharmacy

Pharmacists in institutions supervise the distribution of drugs to patients and provide therapeutic drug monitoring, patient education, formulary services, drug information services, and management services. In addition, pharmacists are assuming greater responsibility for patient education; taking medication histories of admitted patients; monitoring therapeutic drugs; managing the drug regimens of patients; making patient rounds with physicians and nurses to provide drug information; providing pharmacokinetic and therapeutic consultations to physicians, physicians assistants, and advanced practice nurses; and participating in cardiac codes.

Pharmacists serve as consultants to other health-care professionals on drug therapy and conduct in-service education programs for other health professionals on issues related to the use of drugs. In addition, some pharmacists may work in a nuclear pharmacy preparing the various radio pharmaceuticals used in chemotherapy regimens for cancer patients as well as various radioactive testing agents. Decentralization of pharmacy services has expanded the role of institutional pharmacists to a more clinical role. Institutional pharmacists specialize in a variety of areas, including practice management, critical care, ambulatory care, geriatrics, pediatrics, medicine, surgery, oncology, psychiatry, nutrition support, and drug information. Clinical practice with the pharmacist on the floor has dramatically changed the role of the pharmacist to that of a provider of pharmaceutical care.

For more information about institutional pharmacy practice, contact the **American Society of Health-Systems Pharmacists (ASHP),** 7272 Wisconsin Ave., Bethesda, MD 20814; 301-657-3000; fax: 301-652-8278; www.ashp.org.

Pharmaceutical Industry

Many pharmaceutical firms employ pharmacists in research, product development, quality control, clinical research, sales, marketing, management, and several other areas. Pharmacists, as well as other scientists, are responsible for testing and controlling the production of drugs. Once pharmaceuticals have been manufactured, they must be marketed. Pharmacists work in regulatory affairs, dealing with the Food and Drug Administration (FDA), as well as professional affairs, including working with pharmacists, physicians, and other health-care providers and with the general public.

Pharmacists also serve as medical service representatives (sales force of the pharmaceutical industry). These representatives call on physicians, dentists, veterinarians, pharmacists (hospital, community, extended care facilities, and government agencies), and nurses to explain the uses and merits of the products that their firms manufacture.

An expanded area in which there are increasing numbers of pharmacists employed in the pharmaceutical industry is in clinical research, drug information, and product development. The clinical research area utilizes pharmacists to monitor and control clinical research in the field as well as to select research sites.

Another area of the pharmaceutical industry that employs pharmacists is product and consumer information. These pharmacists provide drug information about the companies' products to health-care providers (pharmacists, nurses, physicians, etc.) and to the general public when called upon. They also serve as a resource for the companies' sales and marketing forces. For more information on opportunities in the pharmaceutical industry, contact the **Pharmaceutical Research and Manufacturers of America (PhRMA),** 1100 15th Street NW, Suite 800, Washington, DC 20005; 202-835-3400; fax: 202-835-3414; www.phrma.org.

Government Pharmacy Practice

Many pharmacists work for public health departments on a state or local level as well as for the federal government. In the Food and Drug Administration (FDA), pharmacists work with physicians and other health-care providers in assessing good manufacturing practices and the efficacy of new drug products. In the U.S. Public Health Service, pharmacists are employed as either institutional pharmacy practitioners, administrators, or clinical pharmacists. Pharmacy positions are also available in other governmental agencies, such as the National Institutes of Health where practitioners provide patient-centered pharmaceutical care and also conduct research. There are also opportunities in the armed forces. Each branch of the armed forces has pharmacists that are commissioned officers, and pharmaceutical services are provided in health-care facilities on bases in the U.S. and abroad.

Other pharmacists may participate at the local or state government level as members of licensing boards (State Boards of Pharmacy) as either administrators, inspectors, or board members.

For further information on career opportunities in the federal government, contact the appropriate agency:

U.S. Department of Veterans Affairs, 810 Vermont Avenue NW, Washington, DC 20420; 202-273-8426; fax: 202-273-9067; e-mail: ogden.john@mail.va.gov; www.va.gov.

U.S. Air Force, 89th Medical Group, 1050 West Perimeter, Suite D1-119, Andrews AFB, MD 20762-6600; 301-981-2848; fax: 301-981-4544.

U.S. Army, Walter Reed Army Medical Center, Washington, DC 20307-5001; 202-782-6072; fax: 202-782-0410; e-mail: kent.maneval@na.amedd.army.mil.

U.S. Navy, National Naval Medical Center, Bethesda, MD 20889-5600; 301-295-2120; fax: 301-295-4662.

U.S. Public Health Service (USPHS), 5600 Fishers Lane, Room 9A-05, Rockville, MD 20857; 301-443-7773; fax: 301-549-1171; e-mail: fpaavola@hrsa.ss.

Nuclear Pharmacy

Nuclear pharmacy is a unique specialty area within pharmacy. Individuals who specialize in nuclear pharmacy work with radioactive medications (diagnostic or therapeutic agents) and their preparation. Pharmacists must be certified to work with radioactive materials; generally, a postgraduate course is required. Pharmacy students may take electives in nuclear pharmacy in schools of pharmacy that offer such programs. Postgraduate courses may cover the minimum requirement of 200 hours of work or may include graduate course work leading to a M.S. degree or a Ph.D. Nuclear Pharmacy was the first board-certified specialty recognized by the Board of Pharmaceutical Specialties. For more information on nuclear pharmacy and other pharmacy specialties, contact: **Board of Pharmaceutical Specialties (BPS),** 2215 Constitution Ave. NW, Washington, DC 20037-2985; 202-429-7591; fax: 202-429-6304.

Geriatric Pharmacy Practice

The fastest growing segment of the population is the over-65 group. In 1880, it represented 3 percent of the population; in 1980, it represented 11.3 percent; and by the year 2010, it will constitute 22.5 percent. Geriatric patients have more chronic diseases and therefore use more over-the-counter and prescription medications than any other age group. Because of their medication needs and the unique problems of drug therapy in the elderly, a specialty in geriatric pharmacy practice has been developed. This practitioner provides therapeutic consultation, patient counseling and education, and in-service education to nursing staffs of extended care facilities as well as therapeutic consultations to physicians on the drug therapy of the elderly. Dispensing services are also required for these facilities. This is a new area of practice and one that will offer a rewarding and challenging career.

For more information on geriatric pharmacy or consultant practice, contact: **American Society of Consultant Pharmacists,** 1321 Duke St., Alexandria, VA 22314-3563; 703-739-1300 or 800-355-2727; fax: 703-739-1321 or 800-220-1321; www.ascp.com.

Clinical Practice Specialty Areas

During the past twenty years, a clinical practice of pharmacy has developed that focuses on the provision of rational therapeutics to patients in specific areas. For example, there are pharmacists who are now practicing in specialty areas such as pediatrics, oncology, psychiatry, critical care medicine, pharmacokinetics, geriatrics, pulmonary medicine, and infectious diseases, to mention a few. These practitioners provide services to patients in hospitals and/or clinic situations. In the future, a residency or fellowship will be required in addition to the basic entry-level degree for the profession (Pharm.D.) in order to practice in these specialty areas. The majority of these practitioners today have a Pharm.D. degree and either a specialty residency or fellowship. The specialties that have been recognized for board certification by the Board of Pharmaceutical Specialties are Nutrition Support Pharmacy, Pharmacotherapy, Psychiatry Pharmacy Practice, and Oncology Pharmacy Practice.

For more information on board certification of pharmacists, contact: **Board of Pharmaceutical Specialties (BPS),** 2215 Constitution Ave. NW, Washington, DC 20037-2985; 202-429-7591; fax: 202-429-6304; www.bpsweb.org.

For more information on speciality clinical practice areas in pharmacy, contact: **American College of Clinical Pharmacy (ACCP),** 3101 Broadway, Suite 650, Kansas City, MO 64111; 816-531-2177; fax: 816-531-4990; www.accp.com.

Summary

The profession of pharmacy is a dynamic and changing profession, and should you select pharmacy as your career goal, you will find it rewarding and challenging. Any of the practice areas will provide you with a rewarding and challenging career. This is a partial list of career opportunities; therefore, contact a college, school of pharmacy, or your state pharmacy association for more information on pharmacy career opportunities and pharmacy education.

PART I

The PCAT

ABOUT THE TEST

The Pharmacy College Admission Test (PCAT) is designed to measure the general ability and scientific knowledge of applicants seeking admission to selected schools and colleges of pharmacy. The PCAT is developed and administered by The Psychological Corporation under the auspices of the American Association of Colleges of Pharmacy. The test is generally given four times a year, twice in the fall and twice in the spring. Scores are available about four weeks after the test date.

You may obtain the *Candidate Information Booklet,* which describes the current fee structure and contains an application to take the PCAT, for no charge from The Psychological Corporation. Direct your correspondence and requests for information about the PCAT to:

The Psychological Corporation
PSE Customer Relations-PCAT
19500 Bulverde Road
San Antonio, Texas 78259
800-622-3231 or 210-339-8710
Fax: 888-211-8726 or 210-339-8711
www.tpcweb.com/pse/g-conts0.htm
Monday-Friday, 8:30 a.m.–5:00 p.m. Central Time

It is always advisable to include your name, address, social security number, and the name of the testing program that your letter concerns when writing to The Psychological Corporation.

WHEN IS THE TEST GIVEN

The test is usually given four (4) times a year. Contact The Psychological Corporation for the exact dates as well as the deadlines for submission of applications.

FEES AND SPECIAL SERVICES

The Psychological Corporation accepts fee payments by money order only. Make your money order payable to The Psychological Corporation. If you are applying from outside the United States, you must submit an international money order payable in U.S. dollars.

Your application, along with all the required fees, must be received by the application deadline for the test date for which you are applying. Send your application and fee payments by regular mail to the following address:

The Psychological Corporation
Pharmacy College Admission Test
P.O. Box 91581
Chicago, Illinois 60693

If you need to use overnight courier service to meet the application and fee deadline, please address it to:

The Psychological Corporation
c/o Bank of America
91581 Collections Center Drive
Chicago, Illinois 60693

The following fee schedule is from the 1999–2000 academic year. Please check with The Psychological Corporation for current rates.

FEE SCHEDULE

Test Fee $69.00 (U.S.)

OPTIONAL FEES

Late Application Fee $31.00 (U.S.)
To apply after the regular deadline up to four weeks before the test, you must pay this fee in addition to the test fee.

Special Testing Location Fee $152.00 (U.S.)
To take your test at a location other than a scheduled testing center, you must pay this fee in addition to the test fee.

Standby Registration Fee $39.00 (U.S.)
If you do not preregister to take your test, you must pay this fee in addition to the test fee.

Additional Score Report Fee $16.00 Each (U.S.)
You must pay this fee for each score report beyond the three that your test fee covers and for any requested after you submit your application.

Handscoring Fee $31.00 (U.S.)
To have your electronically scored answer sheet rescored by hand to confirm your reported score, you must pay this additional fee.

TESTING LOCATIONS AND SPECIAL CONSIDERATIONS

Testing centers are located in every state of the United States and throughout Canada. You should contact The Psychological Corporation for exact locations.

Special testing locations for the established testing dates may be arranged for candidates that live more than 150 miles from a scheduled testing center. For candidates whose religious convictions prohibit them to test on a Saturday, a special test date on the Sunday following the scheduled test date may be arranged. Requests for accommodations for candidates with disabilities must be received by The Psychological Corporation by the deadline for application that appears on the back cover of the Candidate Information Booklet.

TEST CONTENT

The PCAT is a multiple-choice test containing approximately 300 questions. Each question has four answer choices listed, only one of which is correct. The answer to any question can be derived independently of any other question.

The student has approximately 3 1/2 hours to complete the examination. This includes a short break halfway through the test.

The PCAT is divided into five areas, and each area is timed separately. During the time for a specific section, you will be allowed to work on that section only. Once you have completed a section and have moved to a new section, you will not be allowed to go back to a previous section. While working on a section, it is advisable to answer those questions that are easy for you, then go back and answer those that are more difficult.

The personal score report that you receive provides you with a total score, scaled score, and the percentile score. The scale ranges from approximately 100 to 300 with a mean of 200 (i.e., a scaled score of 200 is equivalent to the 50th percentile).

CONTENT AREAS

Verbal Ability Section—This section measures general, nonscientific word knowledge using antonyms and analogies. There are approximately 50 questions.

Quantitative Ability Section—This section measures skills in arithmetic processes, including fractions, decimals, percentages, and the ability to reason through and understand quantitative concepts and relationships, including applications of algebra (but not of trigonometry or calculus). There are approximately 65 questions.

Biology Section—This section measures your knowledge of the principles and concepts of basic biology, with a major emphasis on human biology. There are approximately 50 questions.

Chemistry Section—This section measures your knowledge of principles and concepts of inorganic and elementary organic chemistry. There are approximately 60 questions.

Reading Comprehension Section—This section measures your ability to comprehend, analyze, and interpret reading passages on scientific topics. There are approximately 45 questions.

PART II

Practice Tests in PCAT Areas

This chapter includes sample questions in each of the five PCAT content areas. The questions are presented as follows:

Test 1: Verbal Ability	100 questions
Test 2: Quantitative Ability	100 questions
Test 3: Biology	75 questions
Test 4: Chemistry	100 questions
Test 5: Reading Comprehension	43 questions

An answer key and explanatory answers are provided after the last test question.

Answer Sheet

Test 1: Verbal Ability

1. Ⓐ Ⓑ Ⓒ Ⓓ
2. Ⓐ Ⓑ Ⓒ Ⓓ
3. Ⓐ Ⓑ Ⓒ Ⓓ
4. Ⓐ Ⓑ Ⓒ Ⓓ
5. Ⓐ Ⓑ Ⓒ Ⓓ
6. Ⓐ Ⓑ Ⓒ Ⓓ
7. Ⓐ Ⓑ Ⓒ Ⓓ
8. Ⓐ Ⓑ Ⓒ Ⓓ
9. Ⓐ Ⓑ Ⓒ Ⓓ
10. Ⓐ Ⓑ Ⓒ Ⓓ
11. Ⓐ Ⓑ Ⓒ Ⓓ
12. Ⓐ Ⓑ Ⓒ Ⓓ
13. Ⓐ Ⓑ Ⓒ Ⓓ
14. Ⓐ Ⓑ Ⓒ Ⓓ
15. Ⓐ Ⓑ Ⓒ Ⓓ
16. Ⓐ Ⓑ Ⓒ Ⓓ
17. Ⓐ Ⓑ Ⓒ Ⓓ
18. Ⓐ Ⓑ Ⓒ Ⓓ
19. Ⓐ Ⓑ Ⓒ Ⓓ
20. Ⓐ Ⓑ Ⓒ Ⓓ

21. Ⓐ Ⓑ Ⓒ Ⓓ
22. Ⓐ Ⓑ Ⓒ Ⓓ
23. Ⓐ Ⓑ Ⓒ Ⓓ
24. Ⓐ Ⓑ Ⓒ Ⓓ
25. Ⓐ Ⓑ Ⓒ Ⓓ
26. Ⓐ Ⓑ Ⓒ Ⓓ
27. Ⓐ Ⓑ Ⓒ Ⓓ
28. Ⓐ Ⓑ Ⓒ Ⓓ
29. Ⓐ Ⓑ Ⓒ Ⓓ
30. Ⓐ Ⓑ Ⓒ Ⓓ
31. Ⓐ Ⓑ Ⓒ Ⓓ
32. Ⓐ Ⓑ Ⓒ Ⓓ
33. Ⓐ Ⓑ Ⓒ Ⓓ
34. Ⓐ Ⓑ Ⓒ Ⓓ
35. Ⓐ Ⓑ Ⓒ Ⓓ
36. Ⓐ Ⓑ Ⓒ Ⓓ
37. Ⓐ Ⓑ Ⓒ Ⓓ
38. Ⓐ Ⓑ Ⓒ Ⓓ
39. Ⓐ Ⓑ Ⓒ Ⓓ
40. Ⓐ Ⓑ Ⓒ Ⓓ

41. Ⓐ Ⓑ Ⓒ Ⓓ
42. Ⓐ Ⓑ Ⓒ Ⓓ
43. Ⓐ Ⓑ Ⓒ Ⓓ
44. Ⓐ Ⓑ Ⓒ Ⓓ
45. Ⓐ Ⓑ Ⓒ Ⓓ
46. Ⓐ Ⓑ Ⓒ Ⓓ
47. Ⓐ Ⓑ Ⓒ Ⓓ
48. Ⓐ Ⓑ Ⓒ Ⓓ
49. Ⓐ Ⓑ Ⓒ Ⓓ
50. Ⓐ Ⓑ Ⓒ Ⓓ
51. Ⓐ Ⓑ Ⓒ Ⓓ
52. Ⓐ Ⓑ Ⓒ Ⓓ
53. Ⓐ Ⓑ Ⓒ Ⓓ
54. Ⓐ Ⓑ Ⓒ Ⓓ
55. Ⓐ Ⓑ Ⓒ Ⓓ
56. Ⓐ Ⓑ Ⓒ Ⓓ
57. Ⓐ Ⓑ Ⓒ Ⓓ
58. Ⓐ Ⓑ Ⓒ Ⓓ
59. Ⓐ Ⓑ Ⓒ Ⓓ
60. Ⓐ Ⓑ Ⓒ Ⓓ

61. Ⓐ Ⓑ Ⓒ Ⓓ
62. Ⓐ Ⓑ Ⓒ Ⓓ
63. Ⓐ Ⓑ Ⓒ Ⓓ
64. Ⓐ Ⓑ Ⓒ Ⓓ
65. Ⓐ Ⓑ Ⓒ Ⓓ
66. Ⓐ Ⓑ Ⓒ Ⓓ
67. Ⓐ Ⓑ Ⓒ Ⓓ
68. Ⓐ Ⓑ Ⓒ Ⓓ
69. Ⓐ Ⓑ Ⓒ Ⓓ
70. Ⓐ Ⓑ Ⓒ Ⓓ
71. Ⓐ Ⓑ Ⓒ Ⓓ
72. Ⓐ Ⓑ Ⓒ Ⓓ
73. Ⓐ Ⓑ Ⓒ Ⓓ
74. Ⓐ Ⓑ Ⓒ Ⓓ
75. Ⓐ Ⓑ Ⓒ Ⓓ
76. Ⓐ Ⓑ Ⓒ Ⓓ
77. Ⓐ Ⓑ Ⓒ Ⓓ
78. Ⓐ Ⓑ Ⓒ Ⓓ
79. Ⓐ Ⓑ Ⓒ Ⓓ
80. Ⓐ Ⓑ Ⓒ Ⓓ

81. Ⓐ Ⓑ Ⓒ Ⓓ
82. Ⓐ Ⓑ Ⓒ Ⓓ
83. Ⓐ Ⓑ Ⓒ Ⓓ
84. Ⓐ Ⓑ Ⓒ Ⓓ
85. Ⓐ Ⓑ Ⓒ Ⓓ
86. Ⓐ Ⓑ Ⓒ Ⓓ
87. Ⓐ Ⓑ Ⓒ Ⓓ
88. Ⓐ Ⓑ Ⓒ Ⓓ
89. Ⓐ Ⓑ Ⓒ Ⓓ
90. Ⓐ Ⓑ Ⓒ Ⓓ
91. Ⓐ Ⓑ Ⓒ Ⓓ
92. Ⓐ Ⓑ Ⓒ Ⓓ
93. Ⓐ Ⓑ Ⓒ Ⓓ
94. Ⓐ Ⓑ Ⓒ Ⓓ
95. Ⓐ Ⓑ Ⓒ Ⓓ
96. Ⓐ Ⓑ Ⓒ Ⓓ
97. Ⓐ Ⓑ Ⓒ Ⓓ
98. Ⓐ Ⓑ Ⓒ Ⓓ
99. Ⓐ Ⓑ Ⓒ Ⓓ
100. Ⓐ Ⓑ Ⓒ Ⓓ

Tear Here

Test 1: Verbal Ability

100 Questions—1 Hour, 40 Minutes Directions: For questions 1–50, choose the lettered word that means the same or most nearly the same as the word in capital letters.

1. CARDINAL
   - (A) pivotal
   - (B) secondary
   - (C) optional
   - (D) arbitrary

2. AWAKE
   - (A) arouse
   - (B) sleep
   - (C) drowse
   - (D) supply

3. TACT
   - (A) act
   - (B) diplomacy
   - (C) enactment
   - (D) expert

4. EXPERT
   - (A) amateur
   - (B) feat
   - (C) authority
   - (D) neophyte

5. ACCOUNT
   - (A) bookkeeper
   - (B) count
   - (C) basis
   - (D) statement

6. SEQUELA
   - (A) result
   - (B) end
   - (C) aftereffect
   - (D) primary

7. BULLETIN
   - (A) announcement
   - (B) board
   - (C) newt
   - (D) bullet

8. BRIDLE
   - (A) bridge
   - (B) marry
   - (C) restrain
   - (D) center

9. CONTAMINATE
   - (A) pollute
   - (B) contemplate
   - (C) contain
   - (D) purify

10. DISPLEASURE
   - (A) pique
   - (B) disposal
   - (C) madness
   - (D) bitterness

GO ON TO THE NEXT PAGE

11. EVENTUATE
- (A) end
- (B) entwine
- (C) crease
- (D) ensue

12. MAGNIFICENCE
- (A) fame
- (B) magnifier
- (C) grandiosity
- (D) magnitude

13. UNDULATE
- (A) poll
- (B) slither
- (C) retreat
- (D) retch

14. PARSIMONIOUS
- (A) miserly
- (B) liberal
- (C) conservative
- (D) truest

15. QUIESCENT
- (A) mobile
- (B) running
- (C) dormant
- (D) quick

16. RADIOACTIVITY
- (A) radio
- (B) radiation
- (C) radar
- (D) ion

17. COLLEAGUE
- (A) group
- (B) associate
- (C) student
- (D) relative

18. FLANK
- (A) side
- (B) end
- (C) head
- (D) beef

19. DIPSOMANIAC
- (A) diplomat
- (B) insomniac
- (C) alcoholic
- (D) addict

20. CORSAGE
- (A) butler
- (B) nosegay
- (C) receptionist
- (D) corset

21. CORTEGE
- (A) roadway
- (B) retinue
- (C) line
- (D) lineation

22. JOWL
- (A) head
- (B) pig
- (C) owl
- (D) jaw

23. SURMOUNT
    (A) survey
    (B) conquer
    (C) suspect
    (D) recount

24. PLIABLE
    (A) flexible
    (B) scrupulous
    (C) programmable
    (D) reliable

25. ZEAL
    (A) foolishness
    (B) fervor
    (C) pleasure
    (D) pain

26. TRANSCEND
    (A) overtake
    (B) pass
    (C) exceed
    (D) send

27. SHREWD
    (A) cagey
    (B) odd
    (C) shrinkable
    (D) crooked

28. EXPENDITURE
    (A) credit
    (B) disbursement
    (C) debit
    (D) ovolo

29. EXPEDIENCY
    (A) excellence
    (B) expulsion
    (C) efficiency
    (D) appropriateness

30. BEGUILE
    (A) become
    (B) envy
    (C) deceive
    (D) enrage

31. DEPART
    (A) withdraw
    (B) relieve
    (C) repass
    (D) report

32. DENOUNCE
    (A) eulogize
    (B) impeach
    (C) connote
    (D) express

33. DENUDE
    (A) peel
    (B) cancel
    (C) depart
    (D) depress

34. CIRCUMSCRIBE
    (A) chasten
    (B) circulate
    (C) limit
    (D) launch

GO ON TO THE NEXT PAGE

35. DEVIANT

   (A) aberrant

   (B) normal

   (C) nontitled

   (D) ghostly

36. MELEE

   (A) agreement

   (B) melange

   (C) skirmish

   (D) merger

37. ENIGMA

   (A) enemy

   (B) mystery

   (C) mark

   (D) imprecation

38. PALPABLE

   (A) pulpy

   (B) pristine

   (C) touchable

   (D) tactful

39. RUDIMENTARY

   (A) parcel

   (B) mathematical

   (C) parietal

   (D) basal

40. IMPUGN

   (A) deny

   (B) destroy

   (C) implant

   (D) return

41. VALIDATE

   (A) abrogate

   (B) cancel

   (C) authenticate

   (D) abolish

42. TARIFF

   (A) post

   (B) senior

   (C) goal

   (D) duty

43. WASTREL

   (A) vagrant

   (B) spendthrift

   (C) wrangler

   (D) straggler

44. YAHOO

   (A) yak

   (B) ruffian

   (C) blabber

   (D) chat

45. SUAVE

   (A) bluff

   (B) foolish

   (C) urbane

   (D) urban

46. REMORSELESS

   (A) impenitent

   (B) remorseful

   (C) impatient

   (D) regretful

47. PERSNICKETY

(A)   easy

(B)   pernicious

(C)   chancy

(D)   fastidious

48. PERIMETER

(A)   period

(B)   periphery

(C)   area

(D)   end zone

49. IMPERIOUS

(A)   kindly

(B)   gentle

(C)   considerate

(D)   domineering

50. COMPASSION

(A)   unconcern

(B)   implacability

(C)   relentlessness

(D)   sympathy

Directions: For questions 51–100, choose the lettered word that means the opposite or most nearly the opposite of the word in capital letters.

51. DIFFICULTY

(A)   hardship

(B)   burden

(C)   trouble

(D)   effortlessness

52. IDEALISM

(A)   utopianism

(B)   realism

(C)   romanticism

(D)   perfectionism

53. HYSTERICAL

(A)   overwrought

(B)   calm

(C)   worked up

(D)   crazy

54. WELCOME

(A)   hello

(B)   good-bye

(C)   greeting

(D)   salutation

55. AFFLUENT

(A)   glamorous

(B)   stable

(C)   charitable

(D)   scanty

56. EXTRANEOUS

(A)   alien

(B)   foreign

(C)   extrinsic

(D)   intrinsic

57. VULNERABLE

(A)   reverent

(B)   innocent

(C)   unassailable

(D)   inflated

GO ON TO THE NEXT PAGE

58. TAME
- (A) docile
- (B) submissive
- (C) calm
- (D) fierce

59. MAELSTROM
- (A) whirl
- (B) tranquility
- (C) fury
- (D) storm

60. NEFARIOUS
- (A) corrupt
- (B) degenerate
- (C) respectable
- (D) putrid

61. OPPORTUNE
- (A) suitable
- (B) tardy
- (C) seasonable
- (D) timely

62. DIVERSE
- (A) similar
- (B) definite
- (C) happy
- (D) cooperative

63. QUASH
- (A) abrogate
- (B) dissolve
- (C) initiate
- (D) quell

64. CAUSTIC
- (A) sleepy
- (B) sharp
- (C) unintelligent
- (D) soothing

65. ANIMATION
- (A) rebirth
- (B) evisceration
- (C) evaluation
- (D) revivification

66. REMONSTRATION
- (A) challenge
- (B) acquiescence
- (C) difficulty
- (D) demurral

67. ECLECTIC
- (A) selective
- (B) discriminating
- (C) picky
- (D) homogenous

68. FAMOUS
- (A) undistinguished
- (B) celebrated
- (C) redoubtable
- (D) prestigious

69. GLUTTONOUS
- (A) famished
- (B) rapacious
- (C) abstemious
- (D) ravenous

70. GLOAMING

(A)   evening

(B)   morning

(C)   twilight

(D)   eventide

71. TREPIDATION

(A)   honesty

(B)   fearlessness

(C)   anger

(D)   vigor

72. GLIMPSE

(A)   gander

(B)   glance

(C)   peek

(D)   peer

73. GLOOMY

(A)   bright

(B)   unhappy

(C)   dark

(D)   murky

74. INDOLENT

(A)   opulent

(B)   corpulent

(C)   lazy

(D)   industrious

75. JOVIALITY

(A)   mirth

(B)   hilarity

(C)   melancholy

(D)   jollity

76. SAGE

(A)   savant

(B)   buffoon

(C)   scholar

(D)   wise man

77. LISSOME

(A)   rigid

(B)   supple

(C)   lithe

(D)   limber

78. OBDURATE

(A)   callous

(B)   coldhearted

(C)   tender

(D)   mulish

79. OBSTREPEROUS

(A)   blatant

(B)   timorous

(C)   clamorous

(D)   vociferous

80. VALEDICTION

(A)   epistle

(B)   generosity

(C)   greeting

(D)   insecurity

81. OPEN-AIR

(A)   outside

(B)   inside

(C)   alfresco

(D)   outdoor

GO ON TO THE NEXT PAGE

82. ODIOUS

(A) hateful

(B) sinful

(C) spiteful

(D) inoffensive

83. BUOYANCY

(A) ebullience

(B) effervescence

(C) despondence

(D) exuberance

84. RESCIND

(A) reinstate

(B) cancel

(C) mutilate

(D) recall

85. ENTHRALLED

(A) flimsy

(B) empty

(C) bored

(D) weak

86. SENILE

(A) keen

(B) ancient

(C) senescent

(D) decrepit

87. CHASTISE

(A) cleanse

(B) praise

(C) straighten

(D) reprove

88. TEMERITY

(A) daring

(B) caution

(C) adventurousness

(D) audacity

89. MULTICOLORED

(A) variegated

(B) parti-colored

(C) versicolored

(D) monochromatic

90. MODIFY

(A) change

(B) alter

(C) vary

(D) continue

91. FUROR

(A) frenzy

(B) serenity

(C) stir

(D) whirl

92. CONCILIATE

(A) antagonize

(B) pacify

(C) appease

(D) reconcile

93. DESCENDANT

(A) kin

(B) ancestor

(C) seed

(D) progeny

94. FAIR

    (A)   just

    (B)   equitable

    (C)   unbiased

    (D)   biased

95. LASCIVIOUS

    (A)   lewd

    (B)   libertine

    (C)   puritan

    (D)   salacious

96. ACCESSIBLE

    (A)   remarkable

    (B)   salable

    (C)   unavailable

    (D)   obtainable

97. REBUKE

    (A)   reclaim

    (B)   commend

    (C)   reproach

    (D)   complain

98. MOTLEY

    (A)   hodgepodge

    (B)   uniform

    (C)   jumbled

    (D)   mixed

99. IMPROMPTU

    (A)   unplanned

    (B)   extemporaneous

    (C)   improvisational

    (D)   rehearsed

100. WHIMSICAL

    (A)   vagarious

    (B)   whimsied

    (C)   steadfast

    (D)   capricious

STOP   **If you finish before time is called, you may check your work on this section only. Do not turn to any other section in the test.**

Answer Sheet

Test 2: Quantitative Ability

101. Ⓐ Ⓑ Ⓒ Ⓓ	121. Ⓐ Ⓑ Ⓒ Ⓓ	141. Ⓐ Ⓑ Ⓒ Ⓓ	161. Ⓐ Ⓑ Ⓒ Ⓓ	181. Ⓐ Ⓑ Ⓒ Ⓓ
102. Ⓐ Ⓑ Ⓒ Ⓓ	122. Ⓐ Ⓑ Ⓒ Ⓓ	142. Ⓐ Ⓑ Ⓒ Ⓓ	162. Ⓐ Ⓑ Ⓒ Ⓓ	182. Ⓐ Ⓑ Ⓒ Ⓓ
103. Ⓐ Ⓑ Ⓒ Ⓓ	123. Ⓐ Ⓑ Ⓒ Ⓓ	143. Ⓐ Ⓑ Ⓒ Ⓓ	163. Ⓐ Ⓑ Ⓒ Ⓓ	183. Ⓐ Ⓑ Ⓒ Ⓓ
104. Ⓐ Ⓑ Ⓒ Ⓓ	124. Ⓐ Ⓑ Ⓒ Ⓓ	144. Ⓐ Ⓑ Ⓒ Ⓓ	164. Ⓐ Ⓑ Ⓒ Ⓓ	184. Ⓐ Ⓑ Ⓒ Ⓓ
105. Ⓐ Ⓑ Ⓒ Ⓓ	125. Ⓐ Ⓑ Ⓒ Ⓓ	145. Ⓐ Ⓑ Ⓒ Ⓓ	165. Ⓐ Ⓑ Ⓒ Ⓓ	185. Ⓐ Ⓑ Ⓒ Ⓓ
106. Ⓐ Ⓑ Ⓒ Ⓓ	126. Ⓐ Ⓑ Ⓒ Ⓓ	146. Ⓐ Ⓑ Ⓒ Ⓓ	166. Ⓐ Ⓑ Ⓒ Ⓓ	186. Ⓐ Ⓑ Ⓒ Ⓓ
107. Ⓐ Ⓑ Ⓒ Ⓓ	127. Ⓐ Ⓑ Ⓒ Ⓓ	147. Ⓐ Ⓑ Ⓒ Ⓓ	167. Ⓐ Ⓑ Ⓒ Ⓓ	187. Ⓐ Ⓑ Ⓒ Ⓓ
108. Ⓐ Ⓑ Ⓒ Ⓓ	128. Ⓐ Ⓑ Ⓒ Ⓓ	148. Ⓐ Ⓑ Ⓒ Ⓓ	168. Ⓐ Ⓑ Ⓒ Ⓓ	188. Ⓐ Ⓑ Ⓒ Ⓓ
109. Ⓐ Ⓑ Ⓒ Ⓓ	129. Ⓐ Ⓑ Ⓒ Ⓓ	149. Ⓐ Ⓑ Ⓒ Ⓓ	169. Ⓐ Ⓑ Ⓒ Ⓓ	189. Ⓐ Ⓑ Ⓒ Ⓓ
110. Ⓐ Ⓑ Ⓒ Ⓓ	130. Ⓐ Ⓑ Ⓒ Ⓓ	150. Ⓐ Ⓑ Ⓒ Ⓓ	170. Ⓐ Ⓑ Ⓒ Ⓓ	190. Ⓐ Ⓑ Ⓒ Ⓓ
111. Ⓐ Ⓑ Ⓒ Ⓓ	131. Ⓐ Ⓑ Ⓒ Ⓓ	151. Ⓐ Ⓑ Ⓒ Ⓓ	171. Ⓐ Ⓑ Ⓒ Ⓓ	191. Ⓐ Ⓑ Ⓒ Ⓓ
112. Ⓐ Ⓑ Ⓒ Ⓓ	132. Ⓐ Ⓑ Ⓒ Ⓓ	152. Ⓐ Ⓑ Ⓒ Ⓓ	172. Ⓐ Ⓑ Ⓒ Ⓓ	192. Ⓐ Ⓑ Ⓒ Ⓓ
113. Ⓐ Ⓑ Ⓒ Ⓓ	133. Ⓐ Ⓑ Ⓒ Ⓓ	153. Ⓐ Ⓑ Ⓒ Ⓓ	173. Ⓐ Ⓑ Ⓒ Ⓓ	193. Ⓐ Ⓑ Ⓒ Ⓓ
114. Ⓐ Ⓑ Ⓒ Ⓓ	134. Ⓐ Ⓑ Ⓒ Ⓓ	154. Ⓐ Ⓑ Ⓒ Ⓓ	174. Ⓐ Ⓑ Ⓒ Ⓓ	194. Ⓐ Ⓑ Ⓒ Ⓓ
115. Ⓐ Ⓑ Ⓒ Ⓓ	135. Ⓐ Ⓑ Ⓒ Ⓓ	155. Ⓐ Ⓑ Ⓒ Ⓓ	175. Ⓐ Ⓑ Ⓒ Ⓓ	195. Ⓐ Ⓑ Ⓒ Ⓓ
116. Ⓐ Ⓑ Ⓒ Ⓓ	136. Ⓐ Ⓑ Ⓒ Ⓓ	156. Ⓐ Ⓑ Ⓒ Ⓓ	176. Ⓐ Ⓑ Ⓒ Ⓓ	196. Ⓐ Ⓑ Ⓒ Ⓓ
117. Ⓐ Ⓑ Ⓒ Ⓓ	137. Ⓐ Ⓑ Ⓒ Ⓓ	157. Ⓐ Ⓑ Ⓒ Ⓓ	177. Ⓐ Ⓑ Ⓒ Ⓓ	197. Ⓐ Ⓑ Ⓒ Ⓓ
118. Ⓐ Ⓑ Ⓒ Ⓓ	138. Ⓐ Ⓑ Ⓒ Ⓓ	158. Ⓐ Ⓑ Ⓒ Ⓓ	178. Ⓐ Ⓑ Ⓒ Ⓓ	198. Ⓐ Ⓑ Ⓒ Ⓓ
119. Ⓐ Ⓑ Ⓒ Ⓓ	139. Ⓐ Ⓑ Ⓒ Ⓓ	159. Ⓐ Ⓑ Ⓒ Ⓓ	179. Ⓐ Ⓑ Ⓒ Ⓓ	199. Ⓐ Ⓑ Ⓒ Ⓓ
120. Ⓐ Ⓑ Ⓒ Ⓓ	140. Ⓐ Ⓑ Ⓒ Ⓓ	160. Ⓐ Ⓑ Ⓒ Ⓓ	180. Ⓐ Ⓑ Ⓒ Ⓓ	200. Ⓐ Ⓑ Ⓒ Ⓓ

Tear Here

Test 2: Quantitative Ability

101. $\dfrac{3}{8} + \dfrac{4}{5} =$

(A) $\dfrac{95}{80}$

(B) 1.2

(C) $1\dfrac{7}{40}$

(D) $\dfrac{12}{40}$

102. $0.25 + \dfrac{15}{16} =$

(A) 1.08

(B) $1\dfrac{3}{16}$

(C) 3.75

(D) $\dfrac{24}{16}$

103. $1.30 \times 236 =$

(A) 3.068×10^2

(B) 3068×10^1

(C) 283.2

(D) 29.9×10^2

104. $\log(50 \times 2) =$

(A) $(\log 50) \times (\log 2)$

(B) $(\log 2) \times (10 \log 5)$

(C) $\log 10$

(D) $\log 2 + \log 50$

105. $\log 0.001 =$

(A) 3

(B) 100

(C) -3

(D) $\dfrac{1}{3}$

106. $\sqrt[3]{8} =$

(A) 2^3

(B) $\dfrac{8}{2}$

(C) $8^{\frac{1}{3}}$

(D) $8 \log 3$

107. $\log_{10} 1000 =$

(A) 10

(B) 3

(C) 100

(D) 4

GO ON TO THE NEXT PAGE

108. $2 \times 10^{-2} + 2.3 \times 10^1$

    (A) 2.3×10^2

    (B)   24.0

    (C)   23.01

    (D)   23.1

109. $\dfrac{3}{16} =$

    (A)   25%

    (B) $\dfrac{9}{32}$

    (C)   18.75%

    (D)   33%

110. $\dfrac{(2.3g)}{(10ml)} =$

    (A)   2.3%

    (B)   0.23%

    (C)   23% $\dfrac{wt}{vol}$

    (D) $\dfrac{2.3}{100}$

111. How many liters of a 4% solution can be made from 24 g of a drug?

    (A)   6 liters

    (B)   0.6 liter

    (C)   0.096 liter

    (D)   96 liters

112. How much 0.9% NaCl can be made from 1 liter of an 18% stock solution of NaCl?

    (A)   0.05 liter

    (B)   5.0 liters

    (C)   2.0 liters

    (D)   20 liters

113. What is the percentage of ethanol in a mixture composed of 5 liters of 25%, 2 liters of 50%, and 0.5 liter of 10% ethanol?

    (A)   11.3%

    (B)   50%

    (C)   30.7%

    (D)   22%

114. $\log \sqrt{25}$

    (A) $\dfrac{1}{2}\log 25$

    (B) $\log 25^{\frac{1}{2}}$

    (C) $\log 5$

    (D)   All of the above

115. $\log 25^2$

    (A) $\log 50$

    (B)   5

    (C) $\log 5$

    (D) $2 \log 25$

116. If 1 kg equals 2.2 lb, how many grams are in 1 lb?

    (A)   454.5 g

    (B)   2200 g

    (C)   97.8 g

    (D)   1200 g

117. Subtract 283 ml from 1 liter.

    (A)   217 ml

    (B)   9717 ml

    (C)   717 ml

    (D)   None of the above

118. If 15.43 grains are in 1 g, how many milligrams equals 1 grain?

(A) 0.065 mg

(B) 984.6 mg

(C) 84.57 mg

(D) 64.81 mg

119. $\sqrt[3]{3^6} + \sqrt{2^2} =$

(A) 7

(B) 11

(C) 36

(D) None of the above

120. $\left(\dfrac{2}{3}\right)^2 + 2^{-3} =$

(A) $\dfrac{41}{72}$

(B) $\dfrac{4}{48}$

(C) $\dfrac{2}{24}$

(D) $\dfrac{2}{3}$

121. $10^0 + 10^1 + 10^{-1} =$

(A) 10.1

(B) 101

(C) 11.1

(D) 1.1

122. If $9\,(x°C) = 5(y°F) - 160$, what is 79°F in degrees centigrade?

(A) 23.5°C

(B) 87.1°C

(C) 26.1°C

(D) 174.2°C

123. What is −10°C in degrees Fahrenheit?

(A) 50°F

(B) 14°F

(C) −12.2°F

(D) −10°F

124. If the temperature dropped from 72 to 65°F, by how many degrees centigrade did the temperature change?

(A) 7°C

(B) 13.9°C

(C) 44.6°C

(D) 3.9°C

125. What weight of a particular substance is needed to produce 200 ml of a 1:10,000 solution?

(A) 1 g

(B) 200 mg

(C) 0.02 g

(D) 2 mg

GO ON TO THE NEXT PAGE

Questions 126-130 refer to the following graph.

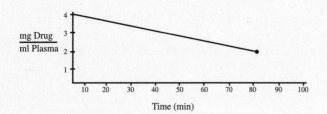

126. At 20 minutes, how much drug remained in the plasma?

    (A)   2 mg/ml

    (B)   There was no change.

    (C)   3.5 mg/ml

    (D)   Cannot be determined from graph

127. At what rate is the drug disappearing from the plasma?

    (A)   2 mg/ml plasma per 60 minutes

    (B)   4 mg/ml plasma per 80 minutes

    (C)   1.5 mg/ml plasma per hour

    (D)   None of the above

128. At 2 hours, what would be the concentration of drug in the plasma?

    (A)   0.5 mg/ml

    (B)   1 mg/ml

    (C)   no drug will remain

    (D)   None of the above

129. If the initial drug concentration had been 8 mg/ml and the rate of disappearance stayed the same, what would have been the drug concentration at 80 minutes?

    (A)   6 mg/ml

    (B)   4 mg/ml

    (C)   2 mg/ml

    (D)   None of the above

130. How long would it take the drug concentration to reach 0 mg/ml if the initial concentration was 4 mg/ml?

    (A)   2 hours

    (B)   200 minutes

    (C)   160 minutes

    (D)   150 minutes

For Questions 131 and 132, find all positive *integers* satisfying the inequality.

131. $4 < 3x - 2 \leq 10$

    (A)   5, 6, 7, 8, 9, 10

    (B)   1, 2, 3

    (C)   3, 4

    (D)   None of the above

132. $\dfrac{7}{x} > 2$, with $x \neq 0$

    (A)   7

    (B)   1, 2, 3

    (C)   2, 7

    (D)   None of the above

133. $\left| -5 \right| - \left| -2 \right| =$

    (A)   -3

    (B)   7

    (C)   3

    (D)   -7

134. $|8| - |14| =$

(A)   6

(B)   -6

(C)   22

(D)   None of the above

135. Solve $|5x + 4| = -3$ for x.

(A) $\dfrac{7}{5}$

(B) $\dfrac{1}{5}$

(C)   2

(D)   None of the above

Questions 136–138 refer to the following diagram.

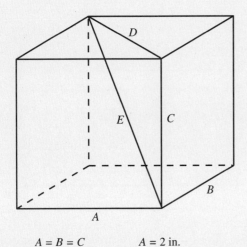

$A = B = C$ $A = 2$ in.

136. What is the length of line D?

(A)   2 in.

(B) $\sqrt{8}$ in.

(C)   4 in.

(D) $\sqrt{5}$ in.

137. What is the area encompassed by lines C, D, and E?

(A) $\sqrt{8}$ in.²

(B) $2\sqrt{3}$ in.²

(C)   2 in.²

(D)   4 in.²

138. What is the total surface area of the cube?

(A)   24 in.²

(B)   16 in.²

(C)   12 in.²

(D)   32 in.²

Questions 139–142 refer to the following diagram.

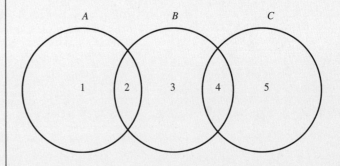

139. The subset _A or B_ encompasses area(s)

(A)   1 and 3

(B)   2

(C)   1, 2, and 3

(D)   1, 2, 3, and 4

140. The subset _A and B_ encompasses area(s)

(A)   1 and 3

(B)   2

(C)   1, 2, and 3

(D)   1, 2, 3, and 4

GO ON TO THE NEXT PAGE

141. The subset _A or C, but not B_ encompasses area(s)

 (A)   1 and 5

 (B)   1, 2, 4, and 5

 (C)   2 and 4

 (D)   1, 4, and 5

142. The subset _B only_ encompasses area(s)

 (A)   1 and 3

 (B)   2, 3, and 4

 (C)   2 and 4

 (D)   3

> Questions 143–145 refer to the following diagrams.

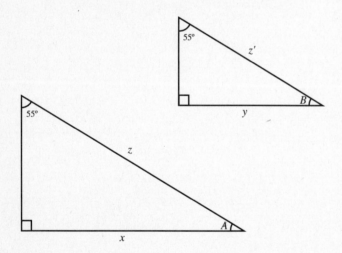

143. If $x = 2y$, what is the ratio of the areas of the two triangles (x:y)?

 (A)   2:1

 (B)   4:1

 (C)   1:2

 (D) $\sqrt{2}$:1

144. How many degrees are there in angle A?

 (A)   60°

 (B)   45°

 (C)   90°

 (D)   35°

145. If $x = 3y$ and $z = 5$, what is z'?

 (A) $\sqrt{5}$

 (B)   3

 (C) $\dfrac{3}{5}$

 (D) $1\dfrac{2}{3}$

> Questions 146 and 147 refer to the following graph.

Percentage of drug assayed as compared to the manufacturer's declared amount.

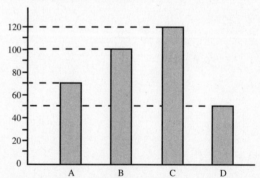

146. If a minimum of 90% of the declared amount of active drug is required by law, which drugs may be used?

 (A)   C only

 (B)   B and C

 (C)   A, B, and C

 (D)   None of the above

147. If the amount of drug declared by the manufacturer was 200 mg, how much drug was present in the drug samples accepted in the previous question?

   (A)   200 mg

   (B)   100 and 120 mg

   (C)   200 and 240 mg

   (D)   None of the above

> Questions 148–150 refer to the following graph.

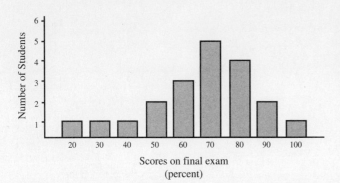

148. What is the mean percent score for the final exam?

   (A)   70%

   (B)   60%

   (C)   66%

   (D)   80%

149. What is the modal score?

   (A)   70%

   (B)   60%

   (C)   66%

   (D)   80%

150. What is the median score?

   (A)   70%

   (B)   60%

   (C)   66%

   (D)   80%

151. If 50 tablets contain 0.625 g of active ingredient, how many tablets can be prepared from 31.25 g of ingredient?

   (A)   2,500 tablets

   (B)   25 tablets

   (C)   625 tablets

   (D)   100 tablets

152. The adult (weight, 150 lb) dose of a drug is 70 μg. Approximately what is the dose for a child weighing 44 lb?

   (A)   200 μg

   (B)   20 μg

   (C)   3 μg

   (D)   None of the above

153. If $x = \dfrac{1}{y}$, what happens to y when x is increased to $2x$?

   (A) y increases by a factor of 2

   (B) y decreases by a factor of $\dfrac{1}{2}$

   (C)   There is no change in y.

   (D) y increases by a factor of 4

154. If $x = 2y$, what happens to y when x is increased to $2x$?

   (A) y increases by a factor of 2

   (B) y decreases by a factor of $\dfrac{1}{2}$

   (C)   There is no change in y.

   (D) y increases by a factor of 4

155. A quantity of drug weighing 24 g is divided into 16 equal parts. How much does each part weigh?

(A) 150 mg

(B) 2666 mg

(C) 0.150 g

(D) 1500 mg

156. If there may be a 10% error in the weight of a tablet, what is the range of acceptable tablet weights when a tablet of 150 g is desired?

(A) 135–150 g

(B) 140–160 g

(C) 130–170 g

(D) 135–165 g

157. If there are 65 mg of elemental iron in 325 mg of ferrous sulfate, what percentage of the tablet weight is due to the iron?

(A) 20%

(B) 2%

(C) 5%

(D) 50%

158. A compound has a maximal solubility of 50 mg/ml. How much is needed to make a 1 liter solution at the maximal concentration?

(A) 5000 mg

(B) 20 g

(C) 1000 mg

(D) 50 g

159. If a graduated cylinder is marked in 5-ml intervals, what is the smallest volume that can be measured with a 10% error?

(A) 5 ml

(B) 50 ml

(C) 100 ml

(D) 10 ml

160. Give the average of the following to the nearest whole number: 61, 50, 100, 50.

(A) 50

(B) 65

(C) 55

(D) Cannot be determined

Questions 161–163 refer to the following graph.

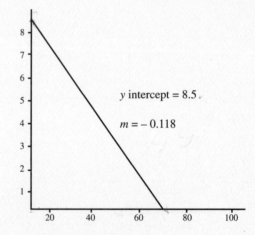

y intercept = 8.5

$m = -0.118$

161. What is the equation for the line?

(A) $y = 8.5 + 0.118x$

(B) $8.5y = 0.118x$

(C) $y = -0.118x + 8.5$

(D) $y = -\dfrac{0.118x}{8.5}$

162. If y equals 6, what is the value of x to the nearest whole number?

    (A)   21

    (B)   40

    (C)   123

    (D)   10

163. If $x = 0$, what is the value of y?

    (A)   0.0

    (B)   0.118

    (C)   8.5

    (D)   None of the above

> Questions 164–166 refer to the following diagram.

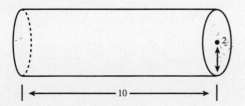

164. What is the volume of the cylinder ($\pi \cong 3.14$)?

    (A)   987 cubic units

    (B)   314 cubic units

    (C)   126 cubic units

    (D)   63 cubic units

165. What is the lateral surface area of the cylinder?

    (A)   987 square units

    (B)   314 square units

    (C)   126 square units

    (D)   63 square units

166. What is the total surface area of the cylinder?

    (A)   314 square units

    (B)   151 square units

    (C)   126 square units

    (D)   135 square units

167. What is the area of the trapezoid when $a = 4$, $b = 2$, and $h = 1$?

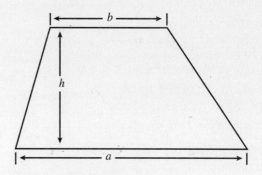

    (A)   4 square units

    (B)   3 square units

    (C)   6 square units

    (D)   8 square units

168. What is the area of the parallelogram when $b = 5$ and $h = 2$?

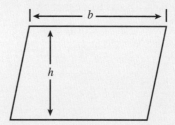

    (A)   5 square units

    (B)   20 square units

    (C)   10 square units

    (D)   2.5 square units

GO ON TO THE NEXT PAGE

169. If $y = 3a + b$ and $x = 3b + a$, find y in terms of x and b.

    (A) $3b + 8x$

    (B) $3b - 8x$

    (C) $3x - 8b$

    (D) $3x + 8b$

170. Given the equation $y = mx + c$, a linear plot of y versus x will yield

    (A)   a slope of m.

    (B)   an ordinate intercept of $1/c$.

    (C)   an abscissa intercept of c.

    (D)   All of the above

171. $\dfrac{7 \div 3}{21 \div 3} =$

    (A) $\dfrac{7}{21}$

    (B) $\dfrac{1}{3}$

    (C) 0.33

    (D)   All of the above

172. Reduce $\dfrac{72}{2880}$ to lowest terms.

    (A) $\dfrac{1}{120}$

    (B) $\dfrac{1}{124}$

    (C) $\dfrac{1}{52}$

    (D) $\dfrac{1}{40}$

173. A prescription calls for 7.5 mg of a drug. How many tablets containing 0.25 mg of the drug are required?

    (A)   30

    (B)   31

    (C)   15

    (D)   17

174. Add $\dfrac{3}{4}$ mg, 0.25 mg, $\dfrac{2}{5}$ mg, and 2.75 mg.

    (A)   5.0 mg

    (B)   4.0 mg

    (C)   4.15 mg

    (D)   5.15 mg

175. Add 0.75 mg, 50 g, and .5 kg.

    (A)   550.00075 g

    (B)   500.75 g

    (C)   0.5575 kg

    (D)   500,575 mg

176. $3\dfrac{1}{8}$ is the same as

    (A) $\dfrac{75}{36}$

    (B) $\dfrac{100}{32}$

    (C) $\dfrac{125}{32}$

    (D) $\dfrac{125}{36}$

177. If 60 mg = 1 grain, then 10% of 360 mg =

(A) 6 grain

(B) 0.6 grain

(C) 0.06 grain

(D) 60 grain

178. $2\sqrt{36} + \dfrac{4\sqrt{28}}{3\sqrt{7}} =$

(A) $14\sqrt{7}$

(B) $12\dfrac{2}{3}$

(C) $13\sqrt{7}$

(D) $14\dfrac{2}{3}$

179. If $A = e^a$, then $1 + A =$

(A) $1 + e^a$

(B) e^a

(C) $\dfrac{1}{e^a}$

(D) $\ln e^a$

180. $7.7 \times 10^0 =$

(A) 0

(B) 0.77

(C) 7.7

(D) 77

181. 1,000,000 can also be expressed as

(A) $1 \times 10^6 \times 10^1$

(B) $1 \times 10^3 \times 10^{-3}$

(C) $1 \times 10^3 \times 10^3$

(D) $1 \times 10^6 \times 10^{-3}$

182. $\sqrt{144 \times 10^4} =$

(A) 2400

(B) 800

(C) 1600

(D) 1200

183. If 1 kg = 2.2 lb, add the following and express the answer in kilograms: 132 lb, 11 lb, and 44 lb.

(A) 85 kg

(B) 88 kg

(C) 98 kg

(D) 58 kg

184. $\left(\dfrac{3}{4}\right)^2 + 3^2 + \sqrt{\dfrac{49}{256}} =$

(A) 27

(B) 10

(C) 29

(D) 30

185. A given line has a slope of –2 and a y intercept $(0, \sqrt{2})$. It can be expressed as the linear equation

(A) $y = -2x$

(B) $y = \sqrt{2} + 2x$

(C) $y = -2x + \sqrt{2}$

(D) $y = 2x$

GO ON TO THE NEXT PAGE

186. Find the value of $\dfrac{250{,}000 \times 0.018}{0.15}$

   (A)   300,000

   (B)   275,000

   (C)   37,000

   (D)   30,000

---

187. What is x if $x^{-3} = \dfrac{1}{27}$?

   (A)   3

   (B) $\dfrac{1}{3}$

   (C)   0.6

   (D)   9

---

188. What is I?

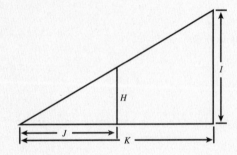

   (A) $\dfrac{KH}{J}$

   (B) $\dfrac{JH}{K}$

   (C) $\dfrac{JK}{H}$

   (D)   None of the above

Questions 189–193 refer to the following statement:

A compound is composed (by weight) of drug A, 20%; drug B, 5%; and drug C, 75%.

189. What amount of drug A is required to make 500 g of the compound?

   (A)   100 g

   (B)   125 g

   (C)   375 g

   (D)   400 g

---

190. What amount of drugs A and B is needed to make 500 g of the compound?

   (A)   100 g

   (B)   125 g

   (C)   375 g

   (D)   400 g

---

191. What amount of drugs B and C is needed to make 500 g of the compound?

   (A)   100 g

   (B)   125 g

   (C)   375 g

   (D)   400 g

---

192. What amount of drugs A, B, and C is needed to make 100 g of the compound?

   (A)   100 g

   (B)   125 g

   (C)   375 g

   (D)   400 g

193. What are the ratios A:B:C as indicated in the formula?

(A) 4:15:1

(B) 4:1:15

(C) 15:1:4

(D) None of the above

---

194. Given that $\dfrac{B-p}{q} = \dfrac{\dfrac{g_a}{M_{-a}}}{\dfrac{g_b}{M_b}}$, find g_b.

(A) $\dfrac{B-p}{q}\dfrac{M_a M_b}{g_a}$

(B) $\dfrac{p-B}{q}\dfrac{M_b g_a}{M_a}$

(C) $\dfrac{q}{B-p}M_b M_a M_a$

(D) $\dfrac{q}{B-p}\dfrac{M_b g_a}{M_a}$

---

195. Consider the following:

Equation 1 $y = 3x + 4$

Equation 2 $y = 3x - 4$

Which best describes equations 1 and 2, respectively?

(A) Slope of +4, y intercept of +3, slope of −4, and y intercept of −3

(B) x intercept of +3, slope of +4, x intercept of −3, and slope of −4

(C) y intercept of +3, slope of +4, y intercept of −3, and slope of −4

(D) Slope of +3, y intercept of +4, slope of +3, and y intercept of −4

---

196. For the following equations, solve for a and b:

$30 = a + 3b - 70$ and $3a + 5b = 100$

(A) $a = -50, b = 50$

(B) $a = 5, b = -5$

(C) $a = -5, b = 5$

(D) $a = 50, b = -50$

---

197. How much medicine would provide a patient with 2 tablespoons twice a day for 10 days? (1 tablespoon = 15 ml)

(A) 300 ml

(B) 600 ml

(C) 450 ml

(D) 900 ml

GO ON TO THE NEXT PAGE

198. If 0.060 of a substance is employed in preparing 125 tablets, how much substance is contained in each tablet?

(A)   390 µg

(B)   420 µg

(C)   450 µg

(D)   480 µg

199. A patient's eye patch measures 12.70 cm across. You have a tape measure in inches. How many inches does the eye patch measure? (1 in = 2.54 cm)

(A)   17 in.

(B)   10 in.

(C)   5 in.

(D)   3 in.

200. $\left(\dfrac{1}{120} \div \dfrac{1}{150}\right) \times 50 =$

(A) $62\dfrac{1}{2}$

(B)   40

(C) $50\dfrac{1}{2}$

(D)   25

S T O P   If you finish before time is called, you may check your work on this section only. Do not turn to any other section in the test.

Answer Sheet

Test 3: Biology

201. Ⓐ Ⓑ Ⓒ Ⓓ   216. Ⓐ Ⓑ Ⓒ Ⓓ   231. Ⓐ Ⓑ Ⓒ Ⓓ   246. Ⓐ Ⓑ Ⓒ Ⓓ   261. Ⓐ Ⓑ Ⓒ Ⓓ

202. Ⓐ Ⓑ Ⓒ Ⓓ   217. Ⓐ Ⓑ Ⓒ Ⓓ   232. Ⓐ Ⓑ Ⓒ Ⓓ   247. Ⓐ Ⓑ Ⓒ Ⓓ   262. Ⓐ Ⓑ Ⓒ Ⓓ

203. Ⓐ Ⓑ Ⓒ Ⓓ   218. Ⓐ Ⓑ Ⓒ Ⓓ   233. Ⓐ Ⓑ Ⓒ Ⓓ   248. Ⓐ Ⓑ Ⓒ Ⓓ   263. Ⓐ Ⓑ Ⓒ Ⓓ

204. Ⓐ Ⓑ Ⓒ Ⓓ   219. Ⓐ Ⓑ Ⓒ Ⓓ   234. Ⓐ Ⓑ Ⓒ Ⓓ   249. Ⓐ Ⓑ Ⓒ Ⓓ   264. Ⓐ Ⓑ Ⓒ Ⓓ

205. Ⓐ Ⓑ Ⓒ Ⓓ   220. Ⓐ Ⓑ Ⓒ Ⓓ   235. Ⓐ Ⓑ Ⓒ Ⓓ   250. Ⓐ Ⓑ Ⓒ Ⓓ   265. Ⓐ Ⓑ Ⓒ Ⓓ

206. Ⓐ Ⓑ Ⓒ Ⓓ   221. Ⓐ Ⓑ Ⓒ Ⓓ   236. Ⓐ Ⓑ Ⓒ Ⓓ   251. Ⓐ Ⓑ Ⓒ Ⓓ   266. Ⓐ Ⓑ Ⓒ Ⓓ

207. Ⓐ Ⓑ Ⓒ Ⓓ   222. Ⓐ Ⓑ Ⓒ Ⓓ   237. Ⓐ Ⓑ Ⓒ Ⓓ   252. Ⓐ Ⓑ Ⓒ Ⓓ   267. Ⓐ Ⓑ Ⓒ Ⓓ

208. Ⓐ Ⓑ Ⓒ Ⓓ   223. Ⓐ Ⓑ Ⓒ Ⓓ   238. Ⓐ Ⓑ Ⓒ Ⓓ   253. Ⓐ Ⓑ Ⓒ Ⓓ   268. Ⓐ Ⓑ Ⓒ Ⓓ

209. Ⓐ Ⓑ Ⓒ Ⓓ   224. Ⓐ Ⓑ Ⓒ Ⓓ   239. Ⓐ Ⓑ Ⓒ Ⓓ   254. Ⓐ Ⓑ Ⓒ Ⓓ   269. Ⓐ Ⓑ Ⓒ Ⓓ

210. Ⓐ Ⓑ Ⓒ Ⓓ   225. Ⓐ Ⓑ Ⓒ Ⓓ   240. Ⓐ Ⓑ Ⓒ Ⓓ   255. Ⓐ Ⓑ Ⓒ Ⓓ   270. Ⓐ Ⓑ Ⓒ Ⓓ

211. Ⓐ Ⓑ Ⓒ Ⓓ   226. Ⓐ Ⓑ Ⓒ Ⓓ   241. Ⓐ Ⓑ Ⓒ Ⓓ   256. Ⓐ Ⓑ Ⓒ Ⓓ   271. Ⓐ Ⓑ Ⓒ Ⓓ

212. Ⓐ Ⓑ Ⓒ Ⓓ   227. Ⓐ Ⓑ Ⓒ Ⓓ   242. Ⓐ Ⓑ Ⓒ Ⓓ   257. Ⓐ Ⓑ Ⓒ Ⓓ   272. Ⓐ Ⓑ Ⓒ Ⓓ

213. Ⓐ Ⓑ Ⓒ Ⓓ   228. Ⓐ Ⓑ Ⓒ Ⓓ   243. Ⓐ Ⓑ Ⓒ Ⓓ   258. Ⓐ Ⓑ Ⓒ Ⓓ   273. Ⓐ Ⓑ Ⓒ Ⓓ

214. Ⓐ Ⓑ Ⓒ Ⓓ   229. Ⓐ Ⓑ Ⓒ Ⓓ   244. Ⓐ Ⓑ Ⓒ Ⓓ   259. Ⓐ Ⓑ Ⓒ Ⓓ   274. Ⓐ Ⓑ Ⓒ Ⓓ

215. Ⓐ Ⓑ Ⓒ Ⓓ   230. Ⓐ Ⓑ Ⓒ Ⓓ   245. Ⓐ Ⓑ Ⓒ Ⓓ   260. Ⓐ Ⓑ Ⓒ Ⓓ   275. Ⓐ Ⓑ Ⓒ Ⓓ

Tear Here

Test 3: Biology

75 QUESTIONS—1 HOUR 40 Minutes Directions: Choose the best answer to each of the following questions.

201. The smallest unit of life is the
    (A) organ.
    (B) organelle.
    (C) cell.
    (D) gene.

202. The organelle primarily responsible for energy production in an aerobic cell is the
    (A) nucleus.
    (B) mitochondria.
    (C) endoplasmic reticulum.
    (D) Golgi apparatus.

203. In humans, brown eyes (*B*) are dominant over blue eyes (*b*). In a cross between two *Bb* individuals, what percentage of offspring will have blue eyes?
    (A) 0%
    (B) 25%
    (C) 75%
    (D) 100%

204. Solutions that cause red blood cells to shrink are called
    (A) isotonic.
    (B) iso-osmotic.
    (C) hypertonic.
    (D) hypotonic.

205. A trace element necessary for normal health of the human body is
    (A) sodium.
    (B) potassium.
    (C) calcium.
    (D) copper.

206. Brown is the dominant color for rats, whereas white is the alternative recessive color. When a homozygous brown rat is crossed with a homozygous white rat, what percentage of the offspring is expected to be brown heterozygous?
    (A) 25%
    (B) 50%
    (C) 75%
    (D) 100%

207. Fat-soluble vitamins include all of the following EXCEPT
    (A) A
    (B) B
    (C) D
    (D) K

GO ON TO THE NEXT PAGE

208. Under basal conditions, the region of the body that receives the greatest blood flow is the

(A) liver.

(B) brain.

(C) bone.

(D) skeletal muscle.

209. Which of the following electrolytes is most abundant in human extracellular fluid?

(A) Sodium

(B) Potassium

(C) Calcium

(D) Magnesium

210. Most nutrients are absorbed by which region of the human gastrointestinal tract?

(A) Stomach

(B) Colon

(C) Small intestine

(D) Large intestine

211. Long-chain fatty acids normally enter the blood system in the form of

(A) cholesterol esters.

(B) free fatty acids.

(C) glycoproteins.

(D) chylomicrons.

212. The most abundant electrolyte in the intracellular fluid of man is

(A) sodium.

(B) potassium.

(C) calcium.

(D) magnesium.

213. In humans, a deficiency in vitamin C (ascorbic acid) is normally associated with

(A) scurvy.

(B) rickets.

(C) pellagra.

(D) beriberi.

214. Squamous epithelium is normally associated with which region of the human body?

(A) Kidney

(B) Lungs

(C) Skin

(D) Pancreas

215. Which of the following statements concerning the structure of a cell is false?

(A) The nucleus of a cell contains DNA and is separated from the surrounding cytoplasm by a nuclear membrane.

(B) The Golgi apparatus, endoplasmic reticulum, and the majority of chromatin are found in the cytoplasm outside the nucleus.

(C) A cell with two complete sets of chromosomes is diploid.

(D) None of the above

216. Which type of muscle will contract most rapidly when stimulated?

(A) Skeletal

(B) Cardiac

(C) Smooth

(D) All muscle types contract at the same rate.

217. Which statement about fatty acids (triglycerides) is true?

(A) Most fats containing unsaturated fatty acids are solids at room temperature, whereas fats containing saturated fatty acids are liquids.

(B) Most fatty acids in nature have an even number of carbon atoms.

(C) Fats yield approximately 50% as much energy as do carbohydrates in humans.

(D) Saturated fatty acids contain one or more double carbon bonds.

218. The nucleic acid responsible for transmitting genetic information from the DNA molecule in the nucleus to the cytoplasm is

(A) transfer RNA.

(B) ribosomal RNA.

(C) messenger RNA.

(D) None of the above

219. The proper sequence for the stages of mitosis is

(A) metaphase, prophase, anaphase, and telophase.

(B) prophase, anaphase, metaphase, and telophase.

(C) prophase, metaphase, telophase, and anaphase.

(D) prophase, metaphase, anaphase, and telophase.

220. Which statement concerning the structure and function of the biological membrane is true?

(A) Biological membranes are primarily composed of protein with a small layer of lipid on both the inner and outer surfaces.

(B) Lipid-soluble compounds tend to diffuse through biological membranes faster than water-soluble ones.

(C) The rate at which lipid-soluble substances pass through biological membranes is determined by the size of the diffusing particle.

(D) All of the above

221. Passive diffusion of substances through biological membranes

(A) requires energy sources such as ATP.

(B) causes a substance to move from a lower to a higher concentration.

(C) can be inhibited by metabolic poisons such as cyanide.

(D) is a major process by which uncharged molecules can move through membranes.

222. The ascending (initial) portion of an action potential observed in a cell is caused by

(A) sodium influx into the cell.

(B) sodium efflux out of the cell.

(C) potassium influx into the cell.

(D) potassium efflux out of the cell.

GO ON TO THE NEXT PAGE

223. The descending portion of an action potential after the initial spike potential in a cell is caused by

(A) sodium influx into the cell.

(B) sodium efflux out of the cell.

(C) potassium influx into the cell.

(D) potassium efflux out of the cell.

224. The normal resting potential of the inner side of a nerve cell relative to the outer side is

(A) 100 mV.

(B) 50 mV.

(C) –50 mV.

(D) –500 mV.

225. Which of the following endogenous substances does not actively aid in the digestion of dietary nutrients?

(A) Pepsin

(B) Insulin

(C) Lactase

(D) Trypsin

226. The organ primarily responsible for detoxifying toxic substances in the blood is the

(A) lung.

(B) kidney.

(C) liver.

(D) pancreas.

227. In humans, the removal of waste products from the blood is one of the primary functions of the

(A) liver.

(B) pancreas.

(C) kidneys.

(D) spleen.

228. Absorption of dietary nutrients can be accomplished by which process?

(A) Active transport

(B) Facilitated diffusion

(C) Passive diffusion

(D) All of the above

229. In humans, bile salts play an important role in enhancing the intestinal absorption of

(A) fatty acids.

(B) glucose.

(C) thiamine.

(D) amino acids.

230. Which of the following sugars is NOT classified as a simple sugar that can be directly absorbed from the digestive tract in man?

(A) Glucose

(B) Fructose

(C) Glycogen

(D) Galactose

231. Which organ of the human body is first affected by a rapid decrease of glucose concentration in the blood?

(A) Brain

(B) Heart

(C) Kidneys

(D) Eyes

232. In humans, night blindness can be due to a diet deficient in

(A) iron.

(B) copper.

(C) vitamin K.

(D) vitamin A.

233. The transport process that does not require the presence of a carrier is

(A) active transport.

(B) passive diffusion.

(C) facilitated diffusion.

(D) None of the above

234. Saturation kinetics are NOT usually observed in which of the following transport processes?

(A) Active transport

(B) Passive diffusion

(C) Facilitated diffusion

(D) Phagocytosis

235. Which theory states that genes exist in individuals as pairs?

(A) The theory of recapitulation

(B) Starling's law

(C) Mendel's law of segregation

(D) The Watson-Crick model

236. Of the following, the element least abundant in the human body is

(A) carbon.

(B) oxygen.

(C) hydrogen.

(D) calcium.

237. Each cell of every organism of a given species contains a characteristic number of chromosomes. How many chromosomes are found in each cell of the human body?

(A) 13

(B) 23

(C) 46

(D) 48

238. In humans, which blood type is known as the universal donor?

(A) O negative

(B) O positive

(C) AB negative

(D) AB positive

239. All of the following substances are known to be neurotransmitters at neuromuscular junctions EXCEPT

(A) epinephrine.

(B) norepinephrine.

(C) acetylcholine.

(D) cholecystokinin.

240. Certain white blood cells are produced in lymphoid tissue such as the spleen, thymus, and lymph nodes. Which of the following white blood cells is produced by lymphoid tissue?

(A) Neutrophils

(B) Monocytes

(C) Eosinophils

(D) None of the above

241. Immunity produced in response to vaccination with some foreign protein (antigen) is known as

(A) actively acquired immunity.

(B) passively acquired immunity.

(C) natural immunity.

(D) cellular immunity.

GO ON TO THE NEXT PAGE

242. The major process by which the kidney removes waste products from the blood is called

(A) tubular secretion.

(B) tubular reabsorption.

(C) glomerular filtration.

(D) tubular sublimation.

243. Stimulation of the human sympathetic nervous system causes all of the following changes in the body EXCEPT

(A) increased heart rate.

(B) increased sweating.

(C) constriction of pupils.

(D) increased blood pressure.

244. Fatigue of a muscle that has contracted many times is primarily caused by an accumulation of

(A) carbon dioxide.

(B) lactic acid.

(C) urea.

(D) sodium chloride.

245. Cell division during which the chromosome number is reduced from diploid to haploid is known as

(A) mitosis.

(B) synapsis.

(C) meiosis.

(D) karyokinesis.

246. The appearance of any individual with respect to a given inherited trait is known as its

(A) genotype.

(B) phenotype.

(C) recessive trait.

(D) heterozygous trait.

247. Which of the following disease states is known to be caused by homozygous recessive genes in an individual?

(A) Sickle cell anemia

(B) Beriberi

(C) Hypertension

(D) Pellagra

248. Intense exercise and training of an athlete can result in which of the following changes?

(A) Increase in the number of muscle fibers

(B) Increased respiratory rate

(C) Increase in the size of muscle fibers

(D) Both A and C

249. During sperm formation, spermatids

(A) develop directly from primary spermatocytes.

(B) contain the diploid number of chromosomes.

(C) develop immediately after the first meiotic division.

(D) develop immediately after the second meiotic division.

250. An individual with type A negative blood can receive blood from which of the following blood types?

(A) O negative

(B) A positive

(C) O positive

(D) All of the above

251. Vestigial organs are the remnants of organs that were functional in some ancestral animal. In man, which organ(s) is NOT vestigial in nature?

(A) Appendix

(B) Wisdom teeth

(C) Coccygeal vertebrae

(D) Pupils of the eyes

252. Which of the following graphs most accurately shows the relation between the substrate (S) and product (P) in a saturated irreversible enzymatic reaction?

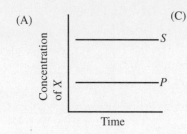

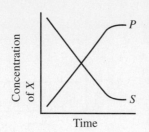

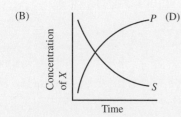

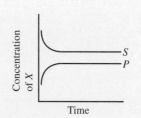

253. Oxygen and carbon dioxide are primarily transported through the blood

(A) dissolved in plasma water.

(B) bound to plasma proteins.

(C) bound to hemoglobin.

(D) None of the above

254. Which of the following statements is false concerning the genetics of man and animals?

(A) Inbreeding is harmful and leads to the production of genetically inferior offspring.

(B) Defective traits can be sex linked.

(C) Outbreeding is the mating of two totally unrelated individuals.

(D) Vigorous inbreeding can result in a high frequency of defects present at birth, termed congenital anomalies.

255. The members of two different species of animals or plants that share the same living space or food source may interact with each other in a positive or negative manner. Which of the following would be a negative interaction?

(A) Parasitism

(B) Commensalism

(C) Pprotocooperation

(D) Mutualism

GO ON TO THE NEXT PAGE

256. Which of the following graphs most accurately shows the relationship between the substrate (*S*) and product (*P*) in a reversible unsaturated enzymatic reaction?

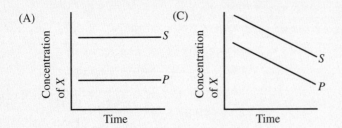

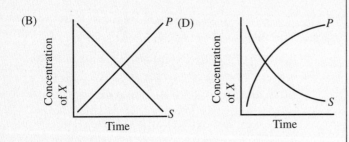

257. Which of the following plasma proteins is most responsible for the osmotic pressure that regulates the water content of the plasma?

(A) Fibrinogen

(B) Albumin

(C) Hemoglobin

(D) Gammaglobulin

258. Which of the following statements is false concerning leukocytes in the human body?

(A) Leukocytes are white blood cells.

(B) Leukocytes move actively by amoeboid movement.

(C) Leukocytes contain hemoglobin.

(D) There is the same number of leukocytes as erythrocytes in plasma.

259. Cells that are very important in the production of antibodies for the immune system are

(A) thrombocytes.

(B) megakaryocytes.

(C) neutrophils.

(D) plasma cells.

260. Which of the following graphs most accurately shows the relationship between the substrate (*S*) and product (*P*) in a saturated reversible enzymatic reaction after treatment with cyanide?

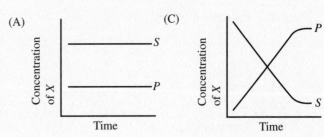

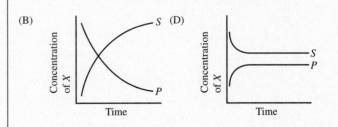

261. The transport of oxygen and carbon dioxide in the blood depends largely on which component of the red blood cell?

(A) Cell wall

(B) Nucleus

(C) Hemoglobin

(D) Cytoplasm

262. The plasma protein most abundant in plasma is

(A) albumin.

(B) globulin.

(C) fibrinogen.

(D) immunoglobin.

263. Which of the following conditions does not increase the number of red blood cells in the human body?

(A) High altitude environment

(B) Low oxygen delivery to the tissues

(C) Increased erythropoietin production

(D) Increased carbon dioxide concentration in the blood

264. Which of the following is NOT associated with heat loss in man?

(A) Sweating

(B) Increased muscle tone

(C) Decreased metabolism

(D) Vasodilation

265. Substances that are actively reabsorbed by the kidney tubules include

(A) urea.

(B) creatinine.

(C) glucose.

(D) All of the above

266. Tissues of the body that are normally involved in regulating the volume of body fluids do NOT include

(A) baroreceptors.

(B) vasomotor center of the brain.

(C) osmoreceptor.

(D) reticular activating system.

267. The structural and functional unit of the nervous system of all multicellular animals is the

(A) axon.

(B) nerve.

(C) neuron.

(D) dendrite.

268. Which of the following statements about the rate of conduction for a nerve impulse is true in humans?

(A) The rate of conduction increases as the diameter of the axon increases.

(B) The rate of conduction is faster in smaller nerve fibers than in larger ones.

(C) Myelin sheaths usually decrease the rate of conduction.

(D) All of the above

269. Which of the following statements concerning the human autonomic nervous system is true?

(A) It controls the voluntary movements of muscles in the limbs.

(B) It is composed of both sympathetic and parasympathetic nerves.

(C) Motor impulses reach the effector organ from the brain or spinal cord by a single neuron.

(D) All of the above

270. In humans, hormones that are derived from amino acids include

(A) prostaglandins.

(B) estradiol.

(C) testosterone.

(D) thyroxine.

GO ON TO THE NEXT PAGE

271. When a skeletal muscle fiber is given a single stimulus, a single twitch with numerous electrical phases is observed. What is the correct order for the phases or periods seen in a skeletal muscle fiber after stimulation?

(A) Contraction, latent, relaxation, refractory

(B) Refractory, contraction, latent, relaxation

(C) Latent, contraction, relaxation, refractory

(D) Latent, refractory, contraction, relaxation

272. Which statement is false concerning the role of hormones in the human body?

(A) Hormones can be secreted by one part of the body, pass through the blood, and act on a target organ in another part of the body.

(B) Neurohormones may pass down axons to the target organ in another part of the body.

(C) Hormones can be derivatives of amino acids, fatty acids, or long peptides.

(D) Hormones usually provide instantaneous control of a bodily function.

273. Hormones for the regulation of the menstrual cycle in women include

(A) progesterone.

(B) vasopressin.

(C) aldosterone.

(D) None of the above

274. In the human eye, the rods located in the retina are responsible for

(A) color vision.

(B) bright light vision.

(C) peripheral vision.

(D) All of the above

275. Which of the following statements is NOT true in reference to the human lymphatic system?

(A) The rate of lymph flow is similar to that of the circulation.

(B) The lymphatic system is an auxiliary system for return of fluid from the tissue spaces to the circulation.

(C) Lymph nodes produce one type of white blood cells, known as lymphocytes.

(D) The lymphatic system plays an important role in the immune process.

STOP If you finish before time is called, you may check your work on this section only. Do not turn to any other section in the test.

Answer Sheet

Test 4: Chemistry

276. Ⓐ Ⓑ Ⓒ Ⓓ	296. Ⓐ Ⓑ Ⓒ Ⓓ	316. Ⓐ Ⓑ Ⓒ Ⓓ	336. Ⓐ Ⓑ Ⓒ Ⓓ	356. Ⓐ Ⓑ Ⓒ Ⓓ
277. Ⓐ Ⓑ Ⓒ Ⓓ	297. Ⓐ Ⓑ Ⓒ Ⓓ	317. Ⓐ Ⓑ Ⓒ Ⓓ	337. Ⓐ Ⓑ Ⓒ Ⓓ	357. Ⓐ Ⓑ Ⓒ Ⓓ
278. Ⓐ Ⓑ Ⓒ Ⓓ	298. Ⓐ Ⓑ Ⓒ Ⓓ	318. Ⓐ Ⓑ Ⓒ Ⓓ	338. Ⓐ Ⓑ Ⓒ Ⓓ	358. Ⓐ Ⓑ Ⓒ Ⓓ
279. Ⓐ Ⓑ Ⓒ Ⓓ	299. Ⓐ Ⓑ Ⓒ Ⓓ	319. Ⓐ Ⓑ Ⓒ Ⓓ	339. Ⓐ Ⓑ Ⓒ Ⓓ	359. Ⓐ Ⓑ Ⓒ Ⓓ
280. Ⓐ Ⓑ Ⓒ Ⓓ	300. Ⓐ Ⓑ Ⓒ Ⓓ	320. Ⓐ Ⓑ Ⓒ Ⓓ	340. Ⓐ Ⓑ Ⓒ Ⓓ	360. Ⓐ Ⓑ Ⓒ Ⓓ
281. Ⓐ Ⓑ Ⓒ Ⓓ	301. Ⓐ Ⓑ Ⓒ Ⓓ	321. Ⓐ Ⓑ Ⓒ Ⓓ	341. Ⓐ Ⓑ Ⓒ Ⓓ	361. Ⓐ Ⓑ Ⓒ Ⓓ
282. Ⓐ Ⓑ Ⓒ Ⓓ	302. Ⓐ Ⓑ Ⓒ Ⓓ	322. Ⓐ Ⓑ Ⓒ Ⓓ	342. Ⓐ Ⓑ Ⓒ Ⓓ	362. Ⓐ Ⓑ Ⓒ Ⓓ
283. Ⓐ Ⓑ Ⓒ Ⓓ	303. Ⓐ Ⓑ Ⓒ Ⓓ	323. Ⓐ Ⓑ Ⓒ Ⓓ	343. Ⓐ Ⓑ Ⓒ Ⓓ	363. Ⓐ Ⓑ Ⓒ Ⓓ
284. Ⓐ Ⓑ Ⓒ Ⓓ	304. Ⓐ Ⓑ Ⓒ Ⓓ	324. Ⓐ Ⓑ Ⓒ Ⓓ	344. Ⓐ Ⓑ Ⓒ Ⓓ	364. Ⓐ Ⓑ Ⓒ Ⓓ
285. Ⓐ Ⓑ Ⓒ Ⓓ	305. Ⓐ Ⓑ Ⓒ Ⓓ	325. Ⓐ Ⓑ Ⓒ Ⓓ	345. Ⓐ Ⓑ Ⓒ Ⓓ	365. Ⓐ Ⓑ Ⓒ Ⓓ
286. Ⓐ Ⓑ Ⓒ Ⓓ	306. Ⓐ Ⓑ Ⓒ Ⓓ	326. Ⓐ Ⓑ Ⓒ Ⓓ	346. Ⓐ Ⓑ Ⓒ Ⓓ	366. Ⓐ Ⓑ Ⓒ Ⓓ
287. Ⓐ Ⓑ Ⓒ Ⓓ	307. Ⓐ Ⓑ Ⓒ Ⓓ	327. Ⓐ Ⓑ Ⓒ Ⓓ	347. Ⓐ Ⓑ Ⓒ Ⓓ	367. Ⓐ Ⓑ Ⓒ Ⓓ
288. Ⓐ Ⓑ Ⓒ Ⓓ	308. Ⓐ Ⓑ Ⓒ Ⓓ	328. Ⓐ Ⓑ Ⓒ Ⓓ	348. Ⓐ Ⓑ Ⓒ Ⓓ	368. Ⓐ Ⓑ Ⓒ Ⓓ
289. Ⓐ Ⓑ Ⓒ Ⓓ	309. Ⓐ Ⓑ Ⓒ Ⓓ	329. Ⓐ Ⓑ Ⓒ Ⓓ	349. Ⓐ Ⓑ Ⓒ Ⓓ	369. Ⓐ Ⓑ Ⓒ Ⓓ
290. Ⓐ Ⓑ Ⓒ Ⓓ	310. Ⓐ Ⓑ Ⓒ Ⓓ	330. Ⓐ Ⓑ Ⓒ Ⓓ	350. Ⓐ Ⓑ Ⓒ Ⓓ	370. Ⓐ Ⓑ Ⓒ Ⓓ
291. Ⓐ Ⓑ Ⓒ Ⓓ	311. Ⓐ Ⓑ Ⓒ Ⓓ	331. Ⓐ Ⓑ Ⓒ Ⓓ	351. Ⓐ Ⓑ Ⓒ Ⓓ	371. Ⓐ Ⓑ Ⓒ Ⓓ
292. Ⓐ Ⓑ Ⓒ Ⓓ	312. Ⓐ Ⓑ Ⓒ Ⓓ	332. Ⓐ Ⓑ Ⓒ Ⓓ	352. Ⓐ Ⓑ Ⓒ Ⓓ	372. Ⓐ Ⓑ Ⓒ Ⓓ
293. Ⓐ Ⓑ Ⓒ Ⓓ	313. Ⓐ Ⓑ Ⓒ Ⓓ	333. Ⓐ Ⓑ Ⓒ Ⓓ	353. Ⓐ Ⓑ Ⓒ Ⓓ	373. Ⓐ Ⓑ Ⓒ Ⓓ
294. Ⓐ Ⓑ Ⓒ Ⓓ	314. Ⓐ Ⓑ Ⓒ Ⓓ	334. Ⓐ Ⓑ Ⓒ Ⓓ	354. Ⓐ Ⓑ Ⓒ Ⓓ	374. Ⓐ Ⓑ Ⓒ Ⓓ
295. Ⓐ Ⓑ Ⓒ Ⓓ	315. Ⓐ Ⓑ Ⓒ Ⓓ	335. Ⓐ Ⓑ Ⓒ Ⓓ	355. Ⓐ Ⓑ Ⓒ Ⓓ	375. Ⓐ Ⓑ Ⓒ Ⓓ

Test 4: Chemistry

100 QUESTIONS—2 HOURS	**Directions:** Choose the best answer to each of the following questions.

276. Alkanes are NOT

   (A) saturated compounds containing carbon and hydrogen.

   (B) formed from sp^3 hybrid orbitals.

   (C) arranged in a straight-chain sequence.

   (D) of the general formula C_nH_{2n}.

277. Regarding phenol,

   (A) a nitro substituent in the ortho position will lower the K_a.

   (B) methyl substituent in the ortho position will lower the K_a.

   (C) methyl substituent in the ortho position will increase the K_a.

   (D) the OH substituent is a meta-directing group.

278. Which of the following is false?

   (A) $pH = \dfrac{(\log 1)}{\left[H^+\right]}$

   (B) $pH + pOH = 14$

   (C) $(H^+)(OH^-) = 10^{-14}$

   (D) $pH - pOH = 14$

279. Calculate the percentage of iron in hematite (Fe_2O_3), given the atomic weights of $Fe = 56$ and $O = 16$.

   (A) 70%

   (B) 2%

   (C) 30%

   (D) 49%

280. How many liters of hydrogen are required to produce 20 liters of ammonia, given the equation $3H_2 + N_2 \rightarrow 2NH_3$?

   (A) 15 liters

   (B) 30 liters

   (C) $33\dfrac{1}{3}$ liters

   (D) 40 liters

281. The volume occupied by the gram-molecular weight of a gas at 0°C and 760 mmHg is

   (A) 1 liter.

   (B) 22.4 liters.

   (C) 32 liters.

   (D) 100 liters.

282. Given the atomic weights of $C = 12$ and $O = 16$, what is the weight of 2 liters of carbon dioxide at standard temperature and pressure?

   (A) 2 g

   (B) 4 g

   (C) 6 g

   (D) 8 g

283. Which of the following hybrid orbitals would carbon form in acetylene?

   (A) sp

   (B) sp^2

   (C) sp^3

   (D) All of the above

284. Which of the following hybrid orbitals would methane and water both form?

(A) *sp*

(B) *sp²*

(C) *sp³*

(D) All of the above

285. The structural formula indicates all of the following EXCEPT

(A) the number of atoms in a molecule.

(B) the gram-molecular volume.

(C) the types of atoms present.

(D) the arrangement of the atom.

286. Pick out the incorrect statement.

(A) Organic compounds may exist as isomers.

(B) Reactions involving organic compounds always proceed faster than those involving inorganic compounds.

(C) Organic compounds are generally soluble in organic solvents.

(D) Organic compounds decompose at relatively lower temperatures than inorganic compounds.

287. When the nucleus of an atom emits a beta particle,

(A) the atomic weight decreases by 4.

(B) the atomic weight increases by 1.

(C) the atomic number increases by 1.

(D) the atomic number stays the same.

288. The conversion of one element into another is termed

(A) transformation.

(B) disintegration.

(C) transmutation.

(D) emanation.

289. All the following are characteristics of gamma rays EXCEPT

(A) high-energy X-rays.

(B) very short wavelength.

(C) deflected by electric fields.

(D) travel at the speed of light.

290. The energy released in nuclear reactions is due to

(A) atomic fusion.

(B) electron capture.

(C) atomic fission.

(D) both fusion and fission.

291. All of the following are alcohols EXCEPT

(A) methanol.

(B) ethanol.

(C) glycerine.

(D) sodium hydroxide.

292. Pick out the incorrect statement concerning hydrogen chloride gas.

(A) It is lighter than air.

(B) It has a pungent smell.

(C) It is soluble in water.

(D) It reacts with ammonia—forming ammonium chloride.

293. All of the following are halogens EXCEPT

(A) bromine.

(B) iodine.

(C) chlorine.

(D) turpentine.

294. The number of equivalents per mole for $HC_2H_3O_2$ is

(A) 1

(B) 2

(C) 3

(D) 4

295. Avogadro's law states that

(A) under identical temperature and pressure, only certain gases contain the same number of molecules.

(B) all gases contain different numbers of molecules, irrespective of pressure or temperature conditions.

(C) only under equal volumes will all gases contain the same number of molecules.

(D) under identical conditions of temperature and pressure, equal volumes of all gases contain the same number of molecules.

296. There are how many different configurations for 2-chlorobutane?

(A) 8

(B) 1

(C) 2

(D) 6

297. The absolute configuration of a chiral molecule may be assigned using the symbols

(A) cis and trans.

(B) R and S.

(C) syn and anti.

(D) alpha and beta.

298. Calculate the amount of sodium chloride crystals needed to supply 100 mg of sodium ions (Na = 23, Cl = 35.5).

(A) 180 mg

(B) 432 mg

(C) 355 mg

(D) 254 mg

299. Calculate the concentration (in milligrams per milliliter) of a solution containing 2 mEq of sodium chloride per milliliter.

(A) 585 mg/ml

(B) 355 mg/ml

(C) 230 mg/ml

(D) 117 mg/ml

300. It has been ordered that Mr. Smith should receive 2 mEq of sodium chloride per kilogram of body weight. Since Mr. Smith weighs 60 kg, how much sodium chloride is needed?

(A) 7 g

(B) 17 g

(C) 27 g

(D) 117 g

GO ON TO THE NEXT PAGE

301. Since the hospital stocks a 0.9% solution of sodium chloride, how much of this solution must be administered to Mr. Smith?

(A) 777 ml

(B) 350 ml

(C) 3500 ml

(D) 7700 ml

302. The pharmacy, however, could only supply a 0.45% solution of sodium chloride. How many liters of this solution must be given to Mr. Smith?

(A) 1.5 liters

(B) 3.0 liters

(C) 4.5 liters

(D) 6.0 liters

303. Electrolytes (e.g., sodium chloride) are important in establishing osmotic pressure; the unit used in measuring osmotic activity is the milliosmol. How many milliosmols of particles does 1 mole of sodium chloride present?

(A) 1 mOsm

(B) 2 mOsm

(C) 3 mOsm

(D) None of the above

304. Osmotic activity is a function of

(A) electrolytes only.

(B) nonelectrolytes only.

(C) strong electrolytes only.

(D) the total number of particles present in solution.

305. If one assumes complete dissociation, how many milliosmols of sodium chloride are in 100 ml of a 0.9% solution?

(A) 2 mOsm

(B) 3 mOsm

(C) 31 mOsm

(D) 45 mOsm

306. Which of the following statements is false?

(A) Hydrogen has one proton.

(B) Hydrogen has one electron in the K shell.

(C) Hydrogen has one neutron in its nucleus.

(D) Hydrogen has an atomic number and an atomic weight of 1.

307. Beryllium has five neutrons and two electrons each in the K and L shell, respectively. Therefore, beryllium has

(A) an atomic weight of 5 and an atomic number of 4.

(B) an atomic weight of 9 and an atomic number of 5.

(C) an atomic weight of 4 and an atomic number of 9.

(D) an atomic weight of 9 and an atomic number of 4.

308. The chemical symbol for mercury is Hg, whereas that for oxygen is 0. If HgO is mercuric oxide, what is mercurous oxide?

(A) HgO_2

(B) Hg_2O

(C) Hg_2O_3

(D) Hg_3O_2

309. HNO_3 is the chemical formula for nitric acid; HNO_2 is the chemical formula for

(A) nitrous acid.

(B) nitronous acid.

(C) nitrate acid.

(D) nitrite acid.

310. The combination of an element A with an element B to form a new compound AB is called a synthetic reaction. The reverse of this reaction is called

(A) single replacement.

(B) synthesis.

(C) decomposition.

(D) double replacement.

311. Pick out the incorrect statement.

(A) Oxidation is associated with the loss of electrons.

(B) Oxidation-reduction reactions involve the loss and gain of electrons.

(C) The oxidized particle (atom) shows a decrease in valence number.

(D) Reduction involves the gain of electrons.

312. You are given the equation $ABC_3 \rightarrow AB + C_2$. The balanced equation is

(A) $2ABC_3 \rightarrow AB + 3C_2$

(B) $ABC_3 \rightarrow AB + C_2$

(C) $2ABC_3 \rightarrow 2AB + 3C_2$

(D) $3ABC_3 \rightarrow 3AB + 3C_2$

313. A molecule of oxygen contains two atoms of oxygen. How many atoms of oxygen does a molecule of ozone contain?

(A) Two

(B) Four

(C) One

(D) Three

314. Which statement is false?

(A) Oxygen burns by itself.

(B) Oxygen is an odorless and colorless gas.

(C) Oxygen supports combustion.

(D) Air contains about 20% oxygen.

315. Hydrogen peroxide decomposes to yield

(A) two molecules of water and two molecules of oxygen.

(B) one molecule of water and one molecule of oxygen.

(C) three molecules of water and two molecules of oxygen.

(D) two molecules of water and one molecule of oxygen.

316. A volumetric flask contains 5000 ml of water. What is the weight of this quantity of water?

(A) 50 g

(B) 500 g

(C) 5000 g

(D) 50,000 g

317. Molarity (M) is best defined as

(A) moles of solute per kiloliter of solution.

(B) moles of solute per kilogram of solution.

(C) moles of solute per 100 ml of solution.

(D) moles of solute per liter of solution.

GO ON TO THE NEXT PAGE

318. A total of 40 g of sodium hydroxide is dissolved in water to give a final volume of 400 ml. What is the molarity of this solution? (Na = 23, O = 16, H = 1)

    (A) 0.25 *M*

    (B) 2.5 *M*

    (C) 25 *M*

    (D) 0.1 *M*

319. How many moles of solute are there in 125 ml of a 5 *M* solution of sodium hydroxide?

    (A) 10.0 mol

    (B) 3.40 mol

    (C) 0.625 mol

    (D) 6.25 mol

320. How much sodium hydroxide is there in 125 ml of a 5 *M* solution of sodium hydroxide?

    (A) 75.0 g

    (B) 62.5 g

    (C) 25.0 g

    (D) 80.5 g

321. What is the molarity of 1 liter of pure water (H$_2$0) ?

    (A) 55 *M*

    (B) 18 *M*

    (C) 19 *M*

    (D) cannot be determined

322. All of the following are colligative properties of solutions EXCEPT the

    (A) boiling point.

    (B) vapor pressure.

    (C) freezing point.

    (D) specific gravity.

323. Given that the hydrogen ion concentration (moles per liter) of a solution is 1.0, what is its pH?

    (A) 0

    (B) 1

    (C) 7

    (D) 14

324. Given the same hydrogen ion concentration (in moles/liter) of 1.0, calculate the pH value of this solution.

    (A) 0

    (B) 1

    (C) 7

    (D) 14

325. The higher the pH of a solution, the

    (A) lower the acidity.

    (B) higher the hydrogen ion concentration.

    (C) lower the basicity.

    (D) stronger the acid.

326. Which of the following statements is false?

    (A) Methane is important in addition reactions.

    (B) Methane is explosive when combined with air.

    (C) Methane is a major component of natural gas.

    (D) Methane is commonly known as marsh gas.

327. All of the following are esters EXCEPT

    (A) ethyl acetate.

    (B) methyl salicylate.

    (C) sodium formate.

    (D) nitroglycerine.

328. Carbohydrates are compounds containing carbon, hydrogen, and oxygen. Which of the following is not a carbohydrate?

(A)   Glucose

(B)   Glyceryl stearate

(C)   Dextran

(D)   Cellulose

329. Pick out the nonsynthetic fiber.

(A)   Cellulose

(B)   Rayon

(C)   Orlon

(D)   Nylon

330. The uncertainty principle, which states that it is impossible to know with exactitude both the momentum and position of an electron simultaneously, is associated with

(A)   Heisenberg.

(B)   Planck.

(C)   de Broglie.

(D)   Bohr.

331. How many quantum numbers are necessary in order to define electronic wave functions?

(A)   4

(B)   3

(C)   2

(D)   1

332. Wolfgang Pauli's exclusion principle states that

(A)   no two electrons in an atom can have the same three quantum numbers.

(B)   no two electrons in an atom can have the same four quantum numbers.

(C)   no two electrons can have the same orbital.

(D)   any two electrons in an atom can have the same four quantum numbers.

333. The electronic distribution in the orbitals of an oxygen atom is

(A) $1s^2 2s^4 2p^2$

(B) $1s^2 2s^2 2p^4$

(C) $1s^2 2s^2 2p^8$

(D) $1s^2 2s^2 2p^6$

334. Carbon has six protons, and its atomic weight is 12. How many electrons and neutrons does it have?

(A)   3 electrons, 9 neutrons

(B)   6 electrons, 6 neutrons

(C)   6 electrons, 12 neutrons

(D)   Cannot be determined from the information given

335. Name the element with the electronic distribution $1s^2 2s^2 2p^2$.

(A)   Helium

(B)   Carbon

(C)   Beryllium

(D)   Oxygen

336. Isotopes are atoms of elements differing only in

(A)   valence.

(B)   the number of electrons.

(C)   chemical property.

(D)   mass.

337. Carbon-14 is a commonly used radioisotope in medical research. How many more neutrons does it have compared to natural carbon?

(A)   2

(B)   4

(C)   6

(D)   0

GO ON TO THE NEXT PAGE

338. Pick out the statement about gamma-ray decay that is false.

(A) The number of protons does not change.

(B) It results in a decrease of 4 units of atomic mass.

(C) There is emission of photons.

(D) The number of neutrons does not change.

339. Electromagnetic radiation has a wide spectrum of energies and wavelengths. The angstrom is widely used as a unit to measure wavelength. What does it equal in meters?

(A) 1×10^{-15} m

(B) 1×10^{-9} m

(C) 1×10^{-10} m

(D) 1×10^{-11} m

340. Pyrophosphoric acid is $H_4P_2O_7$. What does the prefix *pyro-* indicate?

(A) Lowest oxidation state

(B) Highest oxidation state

(C) Highest hydrated form

(D) Loss of water

341. Lead (Pb) has many industrial uses. Lead ion exists in two oxidation states, which are

(A) divalent and tetravalent.

(B) monovalent and trivalent.

(C) divalent and pentavalent.

(D) monovalent and divalent.

342. Plaster of paris is made by heating gypsum until it loses three fourths of its water of hydration. What alkaline-earth metal is found in gypsum and plaster of paris?

(A) Phosphorus

(B) Calcium

(C) Magnesium

(D) Barium

343. Hydrogen sulfide (H_2S) can be prepared by the action of an acid on any metallic sulfide. All of the following are characteristics of hydrogen sulfide EXCEPT

(A) colorless gas.

(B) denser than air.

(C) nontoxic.

(D) odor of rotten eggs.

344. What is the common name for the organic acid with the formula CH_3COOH?

(A) Aqua fortis

(B) Muriatic acid

(C) Aqua regia

(D) Vinegar

345. If table salt is sodium chloride, which of the following is the formula for baking soda?

(A) $Na_2B_4O_7$

(B) $MgSO_4$

(C) Na_2CO_3

(D) $NaHCO_3$

346. HOCl is a more powerful oxidizing agent than chlorine. What is HOCl?

(A)   Tincture of iodine

(B)   Chloroform

(C)   Hypochlorous acid

(D)   Brine

347. Alkenes do NOT possess

(A)   a pi bond.

(B)   an alpha bond.

(C)   a double bond.

(D)   a sigma bond.

348. Amino acids are generally represented by the formula RNH_2COOH. What class of organic compounds is represented by $RCONH_2$?

(A)   Amides

(B)   Esters

(C)   Amines

(D)   Azides

349. In chemistry, the suffix -*ase*, as in lipase, denotes

(A)   a carboxyl group.

(B)   a base.

(C)   an enzyme.

(D)   a sugar.

350. A primary alcohol has at least two hydrogens attached to the alcohol carbon. A tertiary alcohol has

(A)   no hydrogens attached to the alcohol carbon.

(B)   only hydrogen attached to the alcohol carbon.

(C)   three hydrogens attached to the alcohol carbon.

(D)   only one hydrogen attached to the alcohol carbon.

351. Which of the formulas below is methyl vinyl ketone?

(A) $CH_3OCH_2CH = CH_2$

(B) $CH_3COCH = CH_2$

(C) $CH_3CH_2CH_2 = COOH$

(D) $CH_3CH_2COCH = CH_2$

352. The incorrect way of naming an organic acid is by

(A)   using the hydrocarbon name of the longest chain.

(B)   designating the carboxyl carbon as carbon number 1.

(C)   changing the suffix from -*ane* to -*anoic*.

(D)   changing the suffix from -*ane* to -*ol*.

353. Name the hydrocarbon, $CH_3(CH_2)_8CH_3$.

(A)   Nonane

(B)   Octane

(C)   Undecane

(D)   Decane

354. Pick out the incorrect statement.

(A)   Atoms connected by single bonds rotate around the bond.

(B)   Atoms in double bonds are not free to rotate.

(C)   Atoms in a ring are free to rotate around their bonds.

(D)   Atoms in triple bonds are not free to rotate.

GO ON TO THE NEXT PAGE

355. Pick out the incorrect statement.

(A) The stability of a carbonium ion is increased by charge dispersal.

(B) A primary carbonium ion forms more easily than a tertiary carbonium ion.

(C) The carbon atom in a carbonium ion has only six electrons.

(D) Carbonium ions can be classified as primary, secondary, or tertiary.

356. With regard to benzene, which one of the following statements is incorrect?

(A) It is a flat (planar) molecule.

(B) It has the formula C_6H_6.

(C) It is a symmetrical molecule.

(D) It has a bond angle of 150°.

357. With regard to the carbonyl carbons of aldehydes and ketones, which one of the following statements is false?

(A) They usually have a bond angle of 120°.

(B) They are oriented such that carbon and oxygen are joined by a double bond.

(C) They are sp^2 hybridized and not planar.

(D) They are connected to three other atoms by sigma bonds.

358. Nucleophilic substitution is commonly encountered in organic chemistry. Select the one statement below that is correct, concerning nucleophilic displacement.

(A) Amines are more reactive than amides.

(B) Acid chlorides are more reactive than alkyl chloride.

(C) Ethers are more reactive than esters.

(D) Saturated carbons are more reactive than acyl carbon.

359. Glycols are

(A) alcohols containing two hydroxyl groups.

(B) alcohols without any hydroxyl group.

(C) aldehydes containing two hydroxyl groups.

(D) ketones containing two hydroxyl groups.

360. The Grignard reagent is very useful in organic chemistry. Pick out the one incorrect statement about it.

(A) Its general name is alkylmagnesium halide.

(B) The magnesium-halogen bond is covalent.

(C) The carbon-magnesium bond is considered covalent.

(D) Its general formula is RMgX.

361. Which is the correct statement?

(A) Optically inactive reactants yield optically active products.

(B) Optically active products are the result of optically inactive reactants.

(C) Optically inactive reactants yield optically inactive products.

(D) The preparation of dissymmetric compounds from symmetric reactants yields no racemic modification.

362. If CH_4 is methane, what is CH_2?

(A) Methanol

(B) Mesyl

(C) Methyl

(D) Methylene

363. The Diels-Alder reaction does NOT involve

(A) a diene and a dienophile.

(B) a product that is six membered.

(C) $\alpha\beta$-unsaturated carbonyl compounds.

(D) electron-releasing groups in the dienophile.

364. Disaccharides are composed of two monosaccharide units. Which of the following is NOT a disaccharide?

(A) Amylose

(B) Lactose

(C) Maltose

(D) Sucrose

365. Which of the following amino acids is simplest in structure?

(A) Arginine

(B) Tyrosine

(C) Glycine

(D) Methionine

366. Aryl halides are compounds containing

(A) halogen attached to a side chain of an aromatic ring.

(B) halogen attached directly to an aromatic ring.

(C) halogen attached directly to a cyclic alkane.

(D) halogen attached to an alkene.

367. Ethylene oxide is best described as an

(A) alkane.

(B) alkene.

(C) aldehyde.

(D) epoxide.

368. Amines may have all of the following formulas EXCEPT

(A) RNH_2

(B) R_3N

(C) RNH

(D) R_2NH

369. Absolute alcohol is

(A) a mixture of 50 parts of alcohol to water.

(B) 80% alcohol.

(C) water-free alcohol.

(D) wood alcohol.

370. Two aromatic rings sharing a pair of carbon atoms are called fused-ring hydrocarbons. The simplest member of this family of compounds is

(A) naphthalene.

(B) phenanthrene.

(C) benzene.

(D) anthracene.

371. CH_3OH is usually known as

(A) menthone.

(B) methanol.

(C) menthol.

(D) mesitol.

372. All the following describes Tollen's reagent EXCEPT

(A) reduction of silver ion to free silver.

(B) oxidation of an aldehyde.

(C) reduction of an acid to aldehyde.

(D) silver ammonia ion.

GO ON TO THE NEXT PAGE

373. In forming ammonia, nitrogen uses

(A) sp orbitals.

(B) sp^1 orbitals.

(C) sp^2 orbitals.

(D) sp^3 orbitals.

374. An acid chloride can be prepared by substitution of the hydroxyl group of a carboxylic acid. The following reagents are commonly used to prepare acid chlorides EXCEPT

(A) thionyl chloride.

(B) ethyl chloride.

(C) phosphorus trichloride.

(D) phosphorus pentachloride.

375. Which is the incorrect statement?

(A) Sucrose is a reducing sugar.

(B) All monosaccharides are reducing sugars.

(C) Glucose is a monosaccharide.

(D) Glucose is a reducing sugar.

STOP If you finish before time is called, you may check your work on this section only. Do not turn to any other section in the test.

Answer Sheet

Test 5: Reading Comprehension

376. Ⓐ Ⓑ Ⓒ Ⓓ   385. Ⓐ Ⓑ Ⓒ Ⓓ   394. Ⓐ Ⓑ Ⓒ Ⓓ   403. Ⓐ Ⓑ Ⓒ Ⓓ   412. Ⓐ Ⓑ Ⓒ Ⓓ

377. Ⓐ Ⓑ Ⓒ Ⓓ   386. Ⓐ Ⓑ Ⓒ Ⓓ   395. Ⓐ Ⓑ Ⓒ Ⓓ   404. Ⓐ Ⓑ Ⓒ Ⓓ   413. Ⓐ Ⓑ Ⓒ Ⓓ

378. Ⓐ Ⓑ Ⓒ Ⓓ   387. Ⓐ Ⓑ Ⓒ Ⓓ   396. Ⓐ Ⓑ Ⓒ Ⓓ   405. Ⓐ Ⓑ Ⓒ Ⓓ   414. Ⓐ Ⓑ Ⓒ Ⓓ

379. Ⓐ Ⓑ Ⓒ Ⓓ   388. Ⓐ Ⓑ Ⓒ Ⓓ   397. Ⓐ Ⓑ Ⓒ Ⓓ   406. Ⓐ Ⓑ Ⓒ Ⓓ   415. Ⓐ Ⓑ Ⓒ Ⓓ

380. Ⓐ Ⓑ Ⓒ Ⓓ   389. Ⓐ Ⓑ Ⓒ Ⓓ   398. Ⓐ Ⓑ Ⓒ Ⓓ   407. Ⓐ Ⓑ Ⓒ Ⓓ   416. Ⓐ Ⓑ Ⓒ Ⓓ

381. Ⓐ Ⓑ Ⓒ Ⓓ   390. Ⓐ Ⓑ Ⓒ Ⓓ   399. Ⓐ Ⓑ Ⓒ Ⓓ   408. Ⓐ Ⓑ Ⓒ Ⓓ   417. Ⓐ Ⓑ Ⓒ Ⓓ

382. Ⓐ Ⓑ Ⓒ Ⓓ   391. Ⓐ Ⓑ Ⓒ Ⓓ   400. Ⓐ Ⓑ Ⓒ Ⓓ   409. Ⓐ Ⓑ Ⓒ Ⓓ   418. Ⓐ Ⓑ Ⓒ Ⓓ

383. Ⓐ Ⓑ Ⓒ Ⓓ   392. Ⓐ Ⓑ Ⓒ Ⓓ   401. Ⓐ Ⓑ Ⓒ Ⓓ   410. Ⓐ Ⓑ Ⓒ Ⓓ

384. Ⓐ Ⓑ Ⓒ Ⓓ   393. Ⓐ Ⓑ Ⓒ Ⓓ   402. Ⓐ Ⓑ Ⓒ Ⓓ   411. Ⓐ Ⓑ Ⓒ Ⓓ

Tear Here

Test 5: Reading Comprehension

43 QUESTIONS—45 Minutes

Directions: Read each of the following passages and choose the best answer to the questions that follow each passage.

Questions 376–379 are based on the following passage.

Before the intravenous administration of a medication, it is essential to check the medication, dose, fluid in which the drug is to be given, and time of administration against the patient's chart.
(5) After this, all the necessary equipment, such as an alcohol or iodophor sponge, a needle, an intravenous board, tape, and the intravenous solution or admixture, should be assembled. The patient should then be identified by his armband
(10) and the procedure explained to the patient to alleviate any apprehension. Venipuncture can then be performed using a needle or catheter that should be checked after insertion to ensure that it is properly placed in the vein and ad-
(15) equately secured to the patient's arm. The patient should be advised not to disturb the venipuncture site. Because the rate of flow of the solution can be affected by numerous variables (gravity, solution viscosity, temperature, and pos-
(20) sibly defective equipment), it should be checked every hour or so, depending on hospital policy. When the rate of flow is critical, such as in pediatric patients or in parenteral nutrition, an infusion pump may be needed to ensure the proper
(25) flow of solution into the patient.

376. Which of the following items is NOT part of the necessary equipment for administering an intravenous medication?

(A) Alcohol sponge or swab

(B) Needle

(C) Intravenous solution

(D) Intramuscular solution

377. Which of the following is a variable that affects the rate of flow of medication?

(A) Solution color

(B) Solution viscosity

(C) Solution smell

(D) Solution particle size

378. On what kinds of patients should an infusion pump be used?

(A) Pediatric patients

(B) Adult patients

(C) Geriatric patients

(D) Comatose patients

379. Before administering an intravenous solution one must check the

(A) time.

(B) medication against the chart.

(C) day.

(D) dose of the intramuscular drug.

GO ON TO THE NEXT PAGE

Questions 380–384 are based on the following passage.

Adrenergic agents, commonly found in appetite suppressants, bronchodilators, central nervous system stimulants, and vasoconstrictors, produce slight pupillary dilation. They have not been
(5) observed to produce any adverse effects in open-angle glaucoma, and the incidence of deleterious effects on angle closure glaucoma after systemic administration has been extremely low. Adrenergic agents such as epinephrine and phe-
(10) nylephrine have been used ocularly to treat open-angle glaucoma. It is important to note, however, that these agents will elevate the intraocular pressure by narrowing the anterior chamber angle when instilled into eyes of angle
(15) closure patients.

General anesthetics producing parasympathetic and sympathetic imbalance may cause pupillary block. To prevent this complication, topical pilocarpine at 1% may be instilled into the
(20) eye 1 hour prior to anesthesia.

380. Adrenergic agents are commonly found in all of the following EXCEPT

(A) bronchodilators.

(B) bronchoconstrictors.

(C) vasoconstrictors.

(D) appetite suppressants.

381. General anesthetics that produce parasympathetic and sympathetic imbalance may cause

(A) pupillary constriction.

(B) pupillary dilation.

(C) pupillary block.

(D) pupillary stimulation.

382. Adrenergic agents may cause _____ in intraocular pressure.

(A) a decrease

(B) an increase

(C) a slight change

(D) no change

383. Which adrenergic agents have been used to treat open-angle glaucoma?

(A) Epinephrine and ACTH

(B) Epinephrine and propranolol

(C) Epinephrine and phenylephrine

(D) Epinephrine and droperidol

384. Pilocarpine administered _____ hour(s) before anesthesia can prevent the pupillary block caused by anesthetics.

(A) 4

(B) 2

(C) $1\frac{1}{2}$

(D) 1

Questions 385–389 are based on the following passage.

There are numerous methods of administering diphenylhydantoin; however, the regimen must be prescribed individually for each patient because of the many variables that influence the
(5) absorption, distribution, metabolism, and excretion of diphenylhydantoin. Ventricular tachycardia usually requires intravenous therapy. There appears to be no indication in this situation for intramuscular injections, because the drug is
(10) slowly and erratically absorbed from the site, besides being very painful. Diphenylhydantoin plasma levels after intramuscular injection may be 25–50% lower than after equivalent oral doses.

(15) Doses of 50–100 mg of diphenylhydantoin, up to a maximum of 1.0 g, may be administered intravenously every 5 minutes, producing only a mild decrease (10–30 mmHg) in systolic blood pressure. Single intravenous doses of 300 mg or more produce a more marked hypotension (20– (20) 45 mmHg) and also lead to subtherapeutic diphenylhydantoin plasma levels within 20–40 minutes. Generally, cardiovascular complications can be avoided with an infusion rate of 20–50 mg/min.

385. Treatment of ventricular tachycardia with diphenylhydantoin usually requires

(A) sublingual therapy.

(B) intramuscular therapy.

(C) intravenous therapy.

(D) subcutaneous therapy.

386. The dose of diphenylhydantoin that may be given intravenously is

(A) 50–70 mg.

(B) 50–80 mg.

(C) 50–100 mg.

(D) 50–120 mg.

387. With which infusion rate can you avoid cardiovascular complications?

(A) 20–50 mg/min

(B) 20–40 mg/min

(C) 20–30 mg/min

(D) 10–50 mg/min

388. At what dose would you expect to see a marked hypotensive effect from diphenylhydantoin?

(A) 100 mg

(B) 200 mg

(C) 250 mg

(D) 300 mg

389. Which of the following is a reason for NOT administering diphenylhydantoin intramuscularly?

(A) The procedure is too expensive.

(B) The drug is erratically absorbed at the site.

(C) The drug is erratically adsorbed at the site.

(D) The drug is too unstable.

Questions 390–394 are based on the following passage.

In open-angle glaucoma a physical blockage occurs within the trabecular meshwork that retards elimination of aqueous humor. The obstruction is presumed to be located between the tra- (5) becular sheet and the episcleral veins, into which the aqueous humor ultimately flows. The impairment of aqueous drainage elevates the intraocular pressure (IOP) to 25–35 mmHg (normal, 10– 20 mmHg), indicating that the obstruction is (10) usually partial. This increase in IOP is sufficient to cause progressive cupping of the optic disk and eventual visual field defects. As the trabecular spaces become more involved, detachment of the cornea and formation of bullae may de- (15) velop. In addition, scotomata (blind spots) may develop. Since visual acuity remains largely unaffected until late in the disease, presence of scotomata must be regarded as a major indication for the institution of medical therapy.

GO ON TO THE NEXT PAGE

390. Open-angle glaucoma is caused by

   (A)   physical blockage.

   (B)   genetics.

   (C)   physical drainage.

   (D)   infection.

391. Normal IOP has a range of

   (A)   10–15 mmHg.

   (B)   10–25 mmHg.

   (C)   10–20 mmHg.

   (D)   10–30 mmHg.

392. Increases in IOP may cause all of the following EXCEPT

   (A)   progressive cupping of the optic disk.

   (B)   visual field defects (over time).

   (C)   immediate changes in visual field.

   (D)   development of scotomas.

393. Impairment of aqueous drainage elevates the IOP to

   (A)   25–30 mmHg.

   (B)   25–35 mmHg.

   (C)   25–40 mmHg.

   (D)   25–45 mmHg.

394. The obstruction in open-angle glaucoma is presumed to be located between

   (A)   the cornea and the iris.

   (B)   the trabecular sheet and the episcleral veins.

   (C)   the trabecular sheet and the cornea.

   (D)   the episcleral veins and the cornea.

Questions 395–399 are based on the following passage.

An unusual reaction to quinidine is syncope. Besides loss of consciousness, these syncopal attacks involve pallor, muscular twitching, and sometimes seizures. When an EKG is obtained
(5) during an attack, the pattern indicates ventricular tachyarrhythmia that apparently critically decreases cerebral perfusion, causing loss of consciousness. The attacks usually terminate spontaneously, but the rare cases of sudden death
(10) attributed to quinidine are thought to be secondary to ventricular arrhythmia. On the other hand, this condition is often observed in patients with coronary artery disease, where sudden death has been reported to occur as a result of
(15) the primary cardiac pathological condition rather than from the drug itself. Syncope may occur at low doses (e.g., 0.8 g/day) and without evidence of allergic reactions. An adverse dose-related effect is hypotension, which may occur
(20) by alpha-adrenergic receptor blockade or by a direct negative inotropic effect on the heart.

395. Which of the following is NOT associated with syncopal attacks?

   (A)   Pallor

   (B)   Muscular twitching

   (C)   Loss of consciousness

   (D)   Itching

396. An adverse dose-related effect of quinidine is

   (A)   hypertension.

   (B)   hypotension.

   (C)   an inotropic effect.

   (D)   diabetes.

397. When an EKG is obtained during an attack, the pattern indicates

    (A)   arrhythmia.

    (B)   ventricular tachyarrhythmia.

    (C)   ventricular flutter.

    (D)   atrial tachyarrhythmia.

398. An unusual reaction to quinidine is

    (A)   ataxia.

    (B)   pallor.

    (C)   syncope.

    (D)   hypotension.

399. Syncope may occur at

    (A)   high doses of quinidine.

    (B)   moderate doses of quinidine.

    (C)   low doses of quinidine.

    (D)   very high doses of quinidine.

Questions 400–404 are based on the following passage.

Many reports have indicated that the tricyclic antidepressants, especially imipramine, may be of benefit in the treatment of MBD in children. However, although most studies have indicated
(5) their superiority over placebos, they are still not as effective as the psychostimulants. Further drawbacks associated with their use include the development of tolerance in some children and numerous deleterious side effects. Side effects
(10) may be somewhat limited by the maximum daily dose approved by the FDA (5 mg/kg per day), but the patient must be regularly examined for autonomic effects, weight loss, gastrointestinal irritation, fine tremors, hyperirritability, and
(15) mood alterations. In addition, the patient should be monitored for more severe effects on the central nervous system, for example, seizures, and the cardiovascular system, but these can usually be avoided if the practitioner adheres to
(20) FDA recommendations. Although the tricyclic antidepressants are helpful in the treatment of MBD in children, their use at this point is experimental and must be accompanied by certain precautions.

400. Which of the following tricyclic antidepressants has been reported to be effective with MBD?

    (A)   Desipramine

    (B)   Imipramine

    (C)   Amitriptyline

    (D)   Doxepin

401. The maximum daily dose of tricyclic antipressants approved by the FDA is

    (A)   5 mg/kg per day.

    (B)   10 mg/kg per day.

    (C)   15 mg/kg per day.

    (D)   20 mg/kg per day.

402. While the tricyclic antidepressants are superior to placebos, they are still not as effective as

    (A)   hypnotics.

    (B)   sedatives.

    (C)   psychostimulants.

    (D)   stimulants.

403. The patient must be monitored for more severe side effects on the central nervous system such as

    (A)   dizziness.

    (B)   seizures.

    (C)   headaches.

    (D)   blindness.

GO ON TO THE NEXT PAGE

404. Another drawback associated with the use of the tricyclics is

(A) the development of addiction.

(B) sedation.

(C) the development of physical addiction.

(D) the development of tolerance.

Questions 405–408 are based on the following passage.

The primary agents in the treatment of MBD are the centrally acting sympathomimetics, for example, methylphenidate, dextroamphetamine, and magnesium pemoline. This therapeutic approach was first used in 1937, but actual defini-
(5) tion and characterization of this indication in pediatric psychopharmacology did not become popular until the late 1960s. Dextroamphetamine was initially used in 1937 and continued
(10) to be the agent of choice until the late 1960s, when methylphenidate usage increased in association with reports of a lower incidence of side effects with the latter drug. It would appear that these reports of the greater safety of meth-
(15) ylphenidate therapy are of questionable clinical significance. Studies attesting to the greater clinical efficacy of methylphenidate over dextroamphetamine have also been carried out by some authorities who prefer the use of the former
(20) drug, while proponents of dextroamphetamine indicate that, in their hands, it has comparable clinical efficacy at a lower cost.

405. The agent of choice in the treatment of MBD until the late 1960s was

(A) amitriptyline.

(B) dextroamphetamine.

(C) methylphenidate.

(D) magnesium pemoline.

406. Which of the following involves the lowest cost in the treatment of MBD?

(A) Dextroamphetamine

(B) Methylphenidate

(C) Amitriptyline

(D) None of the above

407. Which of the following is NOT a primary agent in the treatment of MBD?

(A) Methylphenidate

(B) Magnesium pemoline

(C) Dextroamphetamine

(D) Chlorpromazine

408. Methylphenidate use increased in the late 1960s due to reports of its

(A) lower cost.

(B) decreased risk of addiction.

(C) lower incidence of side effects.

(D) shorter half-life.

Questions 409–413 are based on the following passage.

Procainamide may be considered as an alternative to quinidine in the treatment and prophylaxis of atrial fibrillation. Most patients absorb 75–95% of an oral dose; however, Koch-Weser
(5) estimated that 10% of subjects may absorb 50% or less. The uncertainty concerning the dose absorbed and the lag time for stomach emptying into the small bowel, where the drug is finally absorbed, force the parenteral administra-
(10) tion of procainamide in emergencies. Procainamide may be given intravenously at a rate of 25–50 mg/min. Giardina et al. have intravenously administered 100 mg, up to a maximum of 1 g, every 5 minutes to treat ventricular ar-

(15) rhythmia. This method will produce a minimally effective serum concentration in 15 minutes. Therapy never had to be interrupted because of hypotension or conduction disturbances; however, the investigators had excluded myo-
(20) cardial infarction patients, who are most susceptible to these adverse reactions, from their population.

---

409. Which of the following drugs may be considered as an alternative to quinidine?

(A) Propranolol

(B) Procainamide

(C) Digoxin

(D) Aspirin

---

410. The dosage used by Giardina et al. to treat ventricular arrhythmias was

(A) 100 mg intravenously every 5 minutes.

(B) 100 mg intramuscularly every 5 minutes.

(C) 200 mg intravenously every 5 minutes.

(D) 200 mg intramuscularly every 5 minutes.

---

411. The normal rate of intravenous administration of procainamide is

(A) 25–100 mg/min.

(B) 25–75 mg/min.

(C) 25–125 mg/min.

(D) 25–50 mg/min.

---

412. Most patients absorb what percentage of an oral dose of procainamide?

(A) 65–75%

(B) 65–95%

(C) 75–95%

(D) 55–75%

---

413. Koch-Weser estimates that 10% of the patients will absorb

(A) 50% or less.

(B) 60% or less.

(C) 70% or less.

(D) 80% or less.

Questions 414–418 are based on the following passage.

Corticosteroid-induced glaucoma is well documented. This form of glaucoma is usually painless and involves no ocular findings or visual field defects. The blockage produced probably occurs
(5) in the trabecular meshwork, severely decreasing the outflow of aqueous humor. Systemically or topically administered corticosteroids further hinder outflow, causing a corresponding increase in intraocular pressure. After topical
(10) therapy, a glaucomatous change occurs in the eye instilled with the drug. This ocular hypertensive effect is usually fully reversible within 1 month after discontinuation of steroid therapy. The increase in intraocular pressure is approxi-
(15) mately 10 mmHg for patients with preglaucomatous anterior chambers, and 5 mmHg for normal persons. In some cases, irreversible eye damage occurs if ocular tension persists for 1–2 months or longer. In addition,
(20) cupping of the optic disk and visual field defects may develop a few months after topical administration of corticosteroids has begun. Patients undergoing chronic topical steroid therapy should therefore have a tonometric ex-
(25) amination every 2 months.

GO ON TO THE NEXT PAGE ➤

414. The increase in intraocular pressure is approximately at what level for patients with preglaucomatous anterior chambers?

(A) 5 mmHg

(B) 10 mmHg

(C) 15 mmHg

(D) 20 mmHg

415. The ocular hypertensive effect caused by corticosteroids is usually

(A) irreversible.

(B) fully reversible.

(C) not seen.

(D) partially reversible.

416. Irreversible eye damage may occur if ocular hypertension persists for

(A) 2–4 months.

(B) 1–2 months.

(C) 1–4 months.

(D) 2–6 months.

417. Corticosteroid-induced glaucoma usually does not involve any of the following symptoms EXCEPT

(A) pain.

(B) physical findings in the eye.

(C) cupping of the optic disk.

(D) night blindness.

418. Patients undergoing chronic topical corticosteroid therapy should have a tonometric every

(A) month.

(B) 2 months.

(C) 3 months.

(D) 4 months.

STOP If you finish before time is called, you may check your work on this section only. Do not turn to any other section in the test.

Answer Keys

Test 1: Verbal Ability

1. A	21. B	41. C	61. B	81. B
2. A	22. D	42. D	62. A	82. D
3. B	23. B	43. B	63. C	83. C
4. C	24. A	44. B	64. D	84. A
5. D	25. B	45. C	65. B	85. C
6. A	26. C	46. A	66. B	86. A
7. A	27. A	47. D	67. D	87. B
8. C	28. B	48. B	68. A	88. B
9. A	29. D	49. D	69. C	89. D
10. A	30. C	50. D	70. B	90. D
11. D	31. A	51. D	71. B	91. B
12. C	32. B	52. B	72. D	92. A
13. B	33. A	53. B	73. A	93. B
14. A	34. C	54. B	74. D	94. D
15. C	35. A	55. D	75. C	95. C
16. B	36. C	56. D	76. B	96. C
17. C	37. B	57. C	77. A	97. B
18. A	38. C	58. D	78. C	98. B
19. C	39. D	59. B	79. B	99. D
20. B	40. A	60. C	80. C	100. C

Test 2: Quantitative Ability

101. C	121. C	141. A	161. C	181. C
102. B	122. C	142. D	162. A	182. D
103. A	123. B	143. B	163. C	183. A
104. D	124. D	144. D	164. C	184. B
105. C	125. C	145. D	165. C	185. C
106. C	126. C	146. B	166. B	186. D
107. B	127. C	147. C	167. B	187. A
108. C	128. B	148. C	168. C	188. A
109. C	129. A	149. A	169. C	189. A
110. C	130. C	150. A	170. A	190. B
111. B	131. C	151. A	171. D	191. D
112. D	132. B	152. B	172. D	192. A
113. C	133. C	153. B	173. A	193. B
114. C	134. A	154. A	174. C	194. D
115. D	135. D	155. D	175. A	195. D
116. A	136. B	156. D	176. B	196. A
117. C	137. A	157. A	177. B	197. B
118. D	138. A	158. D	178. D	198. D
119. B	139. D	159. B	179. A	199. C
120. A	140. B	160. B	180. C	200. A

Test 3: Biology

201. C	216. A	231. A	246. B	261. C
202. B	217. B	232. D	247. A	262. A
203. B	218. C	233. B	248. C	263. D
204. C	219. D	234. B	249. D	264. B
205. D	220. B	235. C	250. A	265. C
206. D	221. D	236. D	251. D	266. D
207. B	222. A	237. C	252. C	267. C
208. A	223. D	238. A	253. C	268. A
209. A	224. C	239. D	254. A	269. B
210. C	225. B	240. D	255. A	270. D
211. D	226. C	241. A	256. D	271. C
212. B	227. C	242. C	257. B	272. D
213. A	228. D	243. C	258. C	273. A
214. C	229. A	244. B	259. D	274. C
215. B	230. C	245. C	260. A	275. A

Test 4: Chemistry

276. D	296. C	316. C	336. D	356. D
277. B	297. B	317. D	337. A	357. C
278. B	298. D	318. B	338. B	358. B
279. A	299. D	319. C	339. C	359. A
280. B	300. A	320. C	340. D	360. B
281. B	301. A	321. A	341. A	361. C
282. B	302. A	322. D	342. B	362. D
283. A	303. B	323. A	343. C	363. D
284. C	304. D	324. D	344. D	364. A
285. B	305. C	325. A	345. D	365. C
286. B	306. C	326. A	346. C	366. B
287. C	307. D	327. C	347. B	367. D
288. C	308. B	328. B	348. A	368. C
289. C	309. A	329. A	349. C	369. C
290. D	310. C	330. A	350. A	370. A
291. D	311. C	331. A	351. B	371. B
292. A	312. C	332. B	352. D	372. C
293. D	313. D	333. B	353. D	373. D
294. A	314. A	334. B	354. C	374. B
295. D	315. D	335. B	355. B	375. A

Test 5: Reading Comprehension

376. D	385. C	394. B	403. B	412. C
377. B	386. C	395. D	404. D	413. A
378. A	387. A	396. B	405. B	414. B
379. B	388. D	397. B	406. A	415. B
380. B	389. B	398. C	407. D	416. B
381. C	390. A	399. C	408. C	417. C
382. B	391. C	400. B	409. B	418. B
383. C	392. C	401. A	410. A	
384. D	393. B	402. C	411. D	

Explanatory Answers
Test 1: Verbal Ability

The verbal ability answers include the basic definition of the word and the corresponding correct answer (the word that means either the same or most nearly the same for questions 1-50, and the word that is opposite in meaning for questions 51-100), as well as whether it is a noun (n), a verb (v), or an adjective (a).

1. **The correct answer is (A).**
   CARDINAL (a)—of foremost importance; pivotal. *Pivotal* (a)—to turn on or as if on a pivot.

2. **The correct answer is (A).**
   AWAKE (v)—roused from or as if from sleep. *Arouse* (v)—to awaken from sleep.

3. **The correct answer is (B).**
   TACT (n)—a keen sense of what to do or say in order to maintain good relations with others. *Diplomacy* (n)—the art and practice of conducting negotiations or affairs without arousing hostility.

4. **The correct answer is (C).**
   EXPERT (n)—one who has acquired special skill in or knowledge and mastery of something. *Authority* (n)—an individual recognized for his or her knowledge in a particular area.

5. **The correct answer is (D).**
   ACCOUNT (n)—chronological record of debit and credit entries posted to a ledger page; a statement of transactions during a fiscal period. *Statement* (n)—a summary of a financial account showing the balance due.

6. **The correct answer is (A).**
   SEQUELA (n)—something that follows, especially a pathological condition resulting from a disease. *Result* (n)—the consequence of a particular action.

7. **The correct answer is (A).**
   BULLETIN (n)—a brief public notice issuing from an authoritative source. *Announcement* (n)—a public notification or declaration.

8. **The correct answer is (C).**
   BRIDLE (v)—to curb or control with or as with a bridle. *Restrain* (v)—to curb or keep under control.

9. **The correct answer is (A).**
   CONTAMINATE (v)—to debase by making impure or unclean. *Pollute* (v)—to make physically impure or unclean.

10. **The correct answer is (A).**
    DISPLEASURE (n)—dissatisfaction or annoyance. *Pique* (n)—displeasure; resentment at being slighted.

11. **The correct answer is (D).**
EVENTUATE (v)—to come out finally; to result. *Ensue* (v)—to take place afterward or as a result.

12. **The correct answer is (C).**
MAGNIFICENCE (n)—richness and splendor. *Grandiosity* (n)—magnificence or grandeur.

13. **The correct answer is (B).**
UNDULATE (v)—to move sinuously; to move in waves. *Slither* (v)—to slide on or as if on a loose, gravely surface; to slip or slide like a snake.

14. **The correct answer is (A).**
PARSIMONIOUS (a)—frugal to the point of stinginess. *Miserly* (a)—greedy and stingy.

15. **The correct answer is (C).**
QUIESCENT (a)—becoming quiet; at rest; inactive. *Dormant* (a)—quiet, still, inactive.

16. **The correct answer is (B).**
RADIOACTIVITY (n)—the property possessed by some elements (such as uranium) of spontaneously emitting alpha, beta, and/or gamma rays by the disintegration of atomic nuclei. *Radiation* (n)—the process of emitting radiant energy in the form of waves or particles.

17. **The correct answer is (C).**
COLLEAGUE (n)—a fellow worker or associate. *Associate* (n)—a friend, partner, or fellow worker.

18. **The correct answer is (A).**
FLANK (n)— the side of anything. *Side* (n)—the right or left part of the wall or trunk of the body.

19. **The correct answer is (C).**
DIPSOMANIAC (n)—an individual with an uncontrollable craving for alcoholic beverages. *Alcoholic* (n)—one affected with alcoholism.

20. **The correct answer is (B).**
CORSAGE (n)—an arrangement of flowers to be worn by a woman. *Nosegay* (n)—a small bunch of flowers.

21. **The correct answer is (B).**
CORTEGE (n)—a train of attendants. *Retinue* (n)—a group of retainers or attendants.

22. **The correct answer is (D).**
JOWL (n)—jaw; one of the lateral halves of the mandible; cheek. *Jaw* (n)—either of two bony structures in most vertebrates that border the mouth.

23. **The correct answer is (B).**
SURMOUNT (v)—to surpass; to overcome or conquer. *Conquer* (v)—to overcome or defeat.

24. **The correct answer is (A).**
PLIABLE (a)—supple enough to bend freely or repeatedly without breaking. *Flexible* (a)—capable of being flexed; pliant.

25. The correct answer is (B).

ZEAL (n)—intense enthusiasm, ardor or fervor. *Fervor* (n)—passion or zeal.

26. The correct answer is (C).

TRANSCEND (v)—to rise above or go beyond the limits of. *Exceed* (v)—to extend outside of; to be greater than or superior to; to go beyond a limit.

27. The correct answer is (A).

SHREWD (a)—marked by discerning awareness and hardheaded acumen; given to wily and artful ways of dealing. *Cagey* (a)—hesitant about committing oneself; wary of being trapped or deceived; shrewd.

28. The correct answer is (B).

EXPENDITURE (n)—the act or process of expending; something expended; disbursement; expense. *Disbursement* (n)—the act of paying out; expenditure.

29. The correct answer is (D).

EXPEDIENCE (n)—the quality or state of being suited to the end in view. *Appropriateness* (n)—especially suitable or compatible; fitting.

30. The correct answer is (C).

BEGUILE (v)—to mislead by cheating or tricking; to deceive. *Deceive* (v)—to mislead or delude.

31. The correct answer is (A).

DEPART (v)—to go away; to turn aside; to swerve. *Withdraw* (v)—to take back or away.

32. The correct answer is (B).

DENOUNCE (v)—to pronounce, especially publicly, someone to be blameworthy or evil; to inform against. *Impeach* (v)—to bring an accusation against; to charge with a crime or misdemeanor.

33. The correct answer is (A).

DENUDE (v)—to strip of all covering; to lay bare by erosion. *Peel* (v)—to remove by stripping.

34. The correct answer is (C).

CIRCUMSCRIBE (v)—to encircle encompass or limit. *Limit* (v)—to curb or restrict.

35. The correct answer is (A).

DEVIANT (a)—straying, especially from a standard principle or topic. *Aberrant* (a)—straying from the current or normal way; deviating from the usual or natural kind.

36. The correct answer is (C).

MELEE (n)—a confused struggle; a hand-to-hand fight among several people. *Skirmish* (n)—a minor fight in war, usually incidental to a larger movement; a minor dispute or contest between opposing parties.

37. The correct answer is (B).

ENIGMA (n)—a perplexing, baffling, or inexplicable matter. *Mystery* (n)—something unexplained or unknown.

38. The correct answer is (C).

PALPABLE (a)—capable of being touched or felt; tangible; easily perceptible. *Touchable* (a)—able to be touched or handled.

39. The correct answer is (D).

RUDIMENTARY (a)—consisting in first principles; of a primitive kind. *Basal* (a)—relating to the situation at or forming the base.

40. The correct answer is (A).

IMPUGN (v)—to attack by argument; to oppose or challenge as false or questionable. *Deny* (v)—to refuse.

41. The correct answer is (C).

VALIDATE (v)—to make legally valid; to grant official sanction to by marking. *Authenticate* (v)— to prove or serve to prove the authenticity of.

42. The correct answer is (D).

TARIFF (n)—a schedule of duties imposed on imported or exported goods. *Duty* (n)—a tax on imports.

43. The correct answer is (B).

WASTREL (n)—a person who wastes; a spendthrift. *Spendthrift* (n)—a person who spends money carelessly or wastefully.

44. The correct answer is (B).

YAHOO (n)—a member of a race of brutes in Swift's *Gulliver's Travels* who have the vices of man; an uncouth or rowdy person. *Ruffian* (n)—a brutal person; a bully.

45. The correct answer is (C).

SUAVE (a)—smoothly though often superficially affable and polite; smooth in performance or finish. *Urbane* (a)—notably polite finished in manner; polished; suave.

46. The correct answer is (A).

REMORSELESS (a)—having no remorse; merciless; persistent and indefatigable. *Impenitent* (a)—not penitent.

47. The correct answer is (D).

PERSNICKETY (a)—fussy about small details; having the characteristics of a snob. *Fastidious* (a)—having high and often capricious standards; showing or demanding excessive delicacy or care.

48. The correct answer is (B).

PERIMETER (n)—the boundary of a closed plane figure; outer limits. *Periphery* (n)—the external boundary of a body; essential nature of a thing.

49. The correct answer is (D).

IMPERIOUS (a)—befitting or characteristic of eminent rank or attainments; marked by arrogant assurance; compelling. *Domineering* (a)—masterful; characterized by overbearing control.

50. The correct answer is (D).
COMPASSION (n)—sympathetic understanding of others' distress together with a desire to alleviate it. *Sympathy* (n)—sameness of feeling; affinity between people.

51. The correct answer is (D).
DIFFICULTY (n)—the quality or state of being difficult; something difficult. *Effortlessness* (n)—showing or requiring little or no effort.

52. The correct answer is (B).
IDEALISM (n)—the theory that true reality is in a realm beyond the form and all the phenomena; the practice of forming ideals or living under their influence. *Realism* (n)—concern for fact or reality and rejection of the impractical and visionary.

53. The correct answer is (B).
HYSTERICAL (a)—characterized by unmanageable fear or emotional excess. *Calm* (a)—still; free from agitation, excitement, or disturbance.

54. The correct answer is (B).
WELCOME (n)—a greeting or cordial remark made upon the entrance or arrival of a guest. *Good-bye* (n)—an ending remark made to one who is leaving.

55. The correct answer is (D).
AFFLUENT (a)—flowing freely; plentiful or abundant. *Scanty* (a)—meager or insufficient.

56. The correct answer is (D).
EXTRANEOUS (a)—existing on the outside; not forming an essential part. *Intrinsic* (a)—belonging to the perimeter of something.

57. The correct answer is (C).
VULNERABLE (a)—open to attack or easily hurt. *Unassailable* (a)—cannot be successfully attacked.

58. The correct answer is (D).
TAME (a)—calm or changed from a state of being wild to a domestic state. *Fierce* (a)—hostile in disposition; given to fighting.

59. The correct answer is (B).
MAELSTROM (n)—a violently confused or agitated state of affairs. *Tranquility* (n)—serenity or calmness.

60. The correct answer is (C).
NEFARIOUS (a)—flagrantly wicked or impious. *Respectable* (a)—worthy of esteem.

61. The correct answer is (B).
OPPORTUNE (a)—happening at the right time. *Tardy* (a)—behind time or late.

62. The correct answer is (A).
DIVERSE (a)—different or varied. *Similar* (a)—nearly the same.

63. **The correct answer is (C).**
QUASH (v)—to nullify, suppress summarily and completely. *Initiate* (v)—to bring into practice or use; to introduce.

64. **The correct answer is (D).**
CAUSTIC (a)—corrosive; sarcastic or biting. *Soothing* (a)—calming; allaying or relieving pain.

65. **The correct answer is (B).**
ANIMATION (n)—the act of giving life or spirit to. *Evisceration* (n)—the taking away of vital force.

66. **The correct answer is (B).**
REMONSTRATION (n)—protestation; presentation of reasons for opposition. *Acquiescence* (n)—the act of accepting without objection.

67. **The correct answer is (D).**
ECLECTIC (a)—composed of elements drawn from various sources. *Homogeneous* (a)—of uniform structure throughout.

68. **The correct answer is (A).**
FAMOUS (a)—honored for outstanding achievement; widely known. *Undistinguished* (a)—not marked by any distinction.

69. **The correct answer is (C).**
GLUTTONOUS (a)—excessive in eating or drinking. *Abstemious* (a)—sparing, especially in eating or drinking.

70. **The correct answer is (B).**
GLOAMING (n)—twilight. *Morning* (n)—dawn; the time from sunrise to noon.

71. **The correct answer is (B).**
TREPIDATION (n)—fearful uncertainty; anxiety. *Fearlessness* (n)—bravery or lack of fear.

72. **The correct answer is (D).**
GLIMPSE (v)—to take a brief look. *Peer* (v)—to look searchingly at something.

73. **The correct answer is (A).**
GLOOMY (a)—partially or totally dark; dismally dark. *Bright* (a)—full of light.

74. **The correct answer is (D).**
INDOLENT (a)—disliking or avoiding work. *Industrious* (a)—hardworking or diligent.

75. **The correct answer is (C).**
JOVIALITY (n)—state of being markedly good humored, convivial, merry. *Melancholy* (n)—depression.

76. **The correct answer is (B).**
SAGE (n)—one distinguished for wisdom and sound judgment. *Buffoon* (n)—one who is always clowning.

77. **The correct answer is (A).**
LISSOME (a)—lithe or nimble. *Rigid* (a)—not flexible; stiff and unyielding.

78. **The correct answer is (C).**
OBDURATE (a)—hardened in feelings; resistant to persuasion or softening influences. *Tender* (a)—having a soft or yielding nature.

79. **The correct answer is (B).**
OBSTREPEROUS (a)—unruly; marked by unruliness or aggressiveness. *Timorous* (a)—fearful or timid.

80. **The correct answer is (C).**
VALEDICTION (n)—a good-bye; the act of saying farewell. *Greeting* (n)—a reception or welcome.

81. **The correct answer is (B).**
OPEN-AIR (a)—outdoor. *Inside* (a)—of, relating to, or being on or near the inside.

82. **The correct answer is (D).**
ODIOUS (a)—disgusting, offensive, hateful. *Inoffensive* (a)—causing no harm or annoyance.

83. **The correct answer is (C).**
BUOYANCE (n)—the tendency of a body to float or rise when submerged in a fluid; lightness or resilience of spirit; cheerfulness. *Despondence* (n)—dejection or loss of hope.

84. **The correct answer is (A).**
RESCIND (v)—to revoke or cancel. *Reinstate* (v)—to restore to a former condition.

85. **The correct answer is (C).**
ENTHRALLED (a)—to be held spell bound or to be captivated by something. *Bored* (a)—to find dull and uninteresting.

86. **The correct answer is (A).**
SENILE (a)—exhibiting a loss of mental faculties associated with old age. *Keen* (a)—showing quick and ardent responsiveness.

87. **The correct answer is (B).**
CHASTISE (v)—to punish; to scold or condemn sharply. *Praise* (v)—to commend.

88. **The correct answer is (B).**
TEMERITY (n)—unreasonable or fool-hardy contempt of danger or opposition; rashness; recklessness. *Caution* (n)—wariness; prudent forethought to minimize risk.

89. **The correct answer is (D).**
MULTICOLORED (a)—displaying a variety of colors. *Monochromatic* (a)—of one color.

90. **The correct answer is (D).**
MODIFY (v)—to make changes in. *Continue* (v)—to keep the same; to maintain without interruption.

91. **The correct answer is (B).**
FUROR (n)—fury or rage. *Serenity* (n)—calmness or tranquility.

92. **The correct answer is (A).**
CONCILIATE (v)—to make compatible; to reconcile. *Antagonize* (v)—to incur or provoke the hostility of.

93. **The correct answer is (B).**
DESCENDANT (n)—one descended from another. *Ancestor* (n)—a person from whom one is descended.

94. **The correct answer is (D).**
FAIR (n)—free from bias; equitable. *Biased* (a)—prejudiced.

95. **The correct answer is (C).**
LASCIVIOUS (a)—lewd, lustful. *Puritan* (a)—relating to the Puritans or Puritanism; morally strict.

96. **The correct answer is (C).**
ACCESSIBLE (a)—obtainable. *Unavailable* (a)—not available.

97. **The correct answer is (B).**
REBUKE (v)—to scold or reprimand. *Commend* (v)—to express approval of or to praise.

98. **The correct answer is (B).**
MOTLEY (a)—composed of many colors or many different elements. *Uniform* (a)—not varying; similar in appearance, pattern, or color.

99. **The correct answer is (D).**
IMPROMPTU (a)—on the spur of the moment; improvised; extemporaneous. *Rehearsed* (a)—practiced beforehand.

100. **The correct answer is (C).**
WHIMSICAL (a)—capricious; impulsive. *Steadfast* (a)—immovable; not subject to change.

Explanatory Answers
Test 2: Quantitative Ability

101. The correct answer is (C).

To add or subtract fractions, convert to equivalent fractions with the same least common denominator (LCD):

$$\frac{3}{8}+\frac{4}{5}=\frac{3\times5}{8\times5}+\frac{4\times8}{5\times8}$$

$$=\frac{15}{40}+\frac{32}{40}$$

$$=\frac{47}{40}$$

$$=1\frac{7}{40}$$

102. The correct answer is (B).

To add or subtract arithmetic fractions and decimal fractions, convert to a common base:

$$0.25+\frac{15}{16}=\frac{4}{16}+\frac{15}{16}$$

$$=\frac{19}{16}$$

$$=1\frac{3}{16}$$

or

$$0.25+\frac{15}{16}=0.25+0.9375$$

$$=1.1875$$

103. The correct answer is (A).

The following relations may be used when dealing with scientific notation:

$$10^{0}=1$$

$$10^{-A}=\frac{1}{10^{A}}$$

$$10^{A+B}=10^{A}\times10^{B}$$

$$\frac{10^{A}}{10^{B}}=10^{A-B}$$

$$\left(10^{A}\right)^{B}=10^{AB}$$

Since

$$1.30 = 1.30 \times 10^0$$

and

$$236 = 2.36 \times 10^2$$

we have

$$(1.30 \times 10^0) \times (2.36 \times 10^2) = 3.068 \times 10^{0+2}$$
$$= 3.068 \times 10^2$$

104. The correct answer is (D).

The log of a product equals the sum of the logs of the component numbers:

$$\log (50 \times 2) = \log 50 + \log 2 = \log 2 + \log 50$$

105. The correct answer is (C).

The logs of multiples of 10, for example, 1, 10, 0.1, are integers:

$10^2 = 100$	$\log 100 = 2$
$10^1 = 10$	$\log 10 = 1$
$10^0 = 1$	$\log 1 = 0$
$10^{-1} = 0.1$	$\log 0.1 = -1$
$10^{-2} = 0.01$	$\log 0.01 = -2$
$10^{-3} = 0.001$	$\log 0.001 = -3$

106. The correct answer is (C).

The root of a power is found by dividing the exponent of the power of the index of the root (see the law of exponents in Answer 119):

$$\sqrt[3]{8}$$

8 is the power

1 is the exponent

3 is the root

$$= 8^{\frac{1}{3}}$$

107. The correct answer is (B).

The log of a number is the exponent of the power to which a given base must be raised in order to equal that number; that is, if

$$y = a^x$$

then

$$\log_a y = x$$

Therefore,

$$\log_{10} 1,000 = 3$$

or base 10 raised to the third power equals 1,000.

108. **The correct answer is (C).**

When adding or subtracting in scientific notation, convert to the same exponent, then add the products; the exponent will remain constant:

$$1 \times 10^{-2} = 0.01 \times 10^0$$

and

$$2.3 \times 10^1 = 23 \times 10^0$$

So,

$$(0.01 \times 10^0) + (23 \times 10^0) = 23.01 \times 10^0$$

$$= 23.01$$

109. **The correct answer is (C).**

Percent, written as %, means per hundred. It is a type of ratio and thus has no units. To express a fraction as a percentage, set 100 as the denominator and multiply by 100%:

$$\frac{3}{16} \times 100\% = 0.1875 \times 100\%$$

$$= 18.75\%$$

110. **The correct answer is (C).**

Weight-per-volume measurements are often expressed as percentages. To calculate the percent weight per volume, convert the fraction to a percentage, that is, with a denominator of 100, times 100%:

$$\frac{2.3g}{10ml} = \frac{23g}{100ml}$$

and

$$\frac{23g}{100ml} \times 100\% = 23\% \frac{wt}{vol}$$

111. **The correct answer is (B).**

This problem involves the use of two ratios set equal to one another to form an equation known as a proportion. To solve a proportion, only one number may be unknown, which will be called x. To solve, rearrange the equation such that x remains alone. Given $A:B = C:D$, the following rules may be used:

1. The product of the means equals the product of the extremes: $B \times C = A \times D$.

2. The product of the means divided by one extreme gives the other extreme:

$$\frac{BC}{A} = D$$

3. The product of the extremes divided by one mean gives the other mean:

$$\frac{AD}{B} = C$$

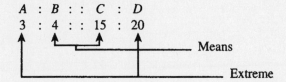

Therefore,

$$4\% \text{ solution} = \frac{4g}{100ml} \text{ (as explained in Answer 110) and}$$

x = number of liters in which 24g will be dissolved.

(Note: 1,000 ml = 1 liter.) Since

$$4\,g : 100\,ml :: 24\,g : x\,ml$$

then

$$\frac{4g}{100ml} = \frac{24g}{x}$$
$$x = \frac{24g \times 100ml}{4g}$$
$$= 600 \text{ ml or } 0.6 \text{ liter}$$

112.   **The correct answer is (D).**

This problem is similar to that of Question 111 in that a proportionality is needed to solve the problem. First determine the total number of grams of NaCl that will be used to make the 0.9% solution:

$$18\% = \frac{18g}{100ml} \times 1,000ml$$

$$= 180g$$

This quantity will be diluted with the final total volume, the unknown x, which should result in a 0.9% solution:

$$0.9\% = \frac{0.9\,g}{100\,ml}$$

and

$$\frac{0.9\%}{100\,ml} = \frac{180\,g}{x\,ml}$$

So,

$$x\,ml = \frac{180g \times 100ml}{0.9g}$$
$$= 20,000 \text{ ml}$$
$$= 20 \text{ liters}$$

113. **The correct answer is (C).**

When one mixes different strengths, the units and types of percent (wt/wt, wt/vol, vol/vol) must be kept constant. Determine the total amount of alcohol in all solutions and the total amount of solution, assuming additivity of volumes on mixing. Then, convert to the desired final ration:

$$25\% \times 5{,}000 \text{ ml} = 1{,}250 \text{ ml}$$

$$50\% \times 2{,}000 \text{ ml} = 1{,}000 \text{ ml}$$

$$10\% \times \frac{50 \text{ ml}}{7{,}500 \text{ ml}} = \frac{50 \text{ ml}}{2{,}300 \text{ ml}} \text{ ethanol}$$

So

$$\frac{2{,}300 \text{ ml of ethanol}}{7{,}500 \text{ ml of solution}} = 0.3067 \cong 30.7\%$$

114. **The correct answer is (C).**

The laws of logarithms are derived from the laws of exponents (see Answer 119). The most commonly used base is 10, although any base may be used.

$$\log (ab) \quad = \quad \log a + \log b$$

$$\log \left(\frac{a}{b}\right) \quad = \quad \log a - \log b$$

$$\log a^n \quad = \quad n \times \log a$$

$$\log a^{\frac{1}{n}} \quad = \quad \log \sqrt[n]{a} = \left(\frac{1}{n}\right) \log a$$

Therefore,

$$\log \sqrt{25} = \frac{1}{2} \log 25 = \frac{(\log 25)}{2}$$

$$= \log 25^{\frac{1}{2}}$$

$$= \log 5$$

115. **The correct answer is (D).**

From previous answers,

$$\log a^n = n \times \log a$$

$$\log 25^2 = 2 \times \log 25$$

116. **The correct answer is (A).**

This problem involves ratios. First convert the common units:

$$1 \text{ kg} = 1{,}000 \text{ g}$$

Then set up the proportionality:

$$\frac{1 \text{ kg}}{2.2 \text{ lb}} = \frac{x}{1 \text{ lb}}$$

$$\frac{1{,}000 \text{g} \times (1 \text{ lb})}{2.2 \text{ lb}} = x$$

$$454.5 \text{ g} = x$$

117. **The correct answer is (C).**

Whenever mathematical procedures are used, all the units must be the same. Therefore,

$$1 \text{ liter} = 1{,}000 \text{ ml}$$

and

$$1{,}000 \text{ ml} - 283 \text{ ml} = 717 \text{ ml}$$

118. **The correct answer is (D).**

(See Answer 111 and 116.)

$$\text{Since } 1 \text{ g} = 1{,}000 \text{ mg}$$

we have

$$\frac{15.43 \text{ grains}}{1{,}000 \text{ mg}} = \frac{1 \text{ grain}}{x \text{ mg}}$$

$$x \text{ mg} = \frac{1 \text{ grain} \times 1{,}000 \text{ mg}}{15.43 \text{ grains}}$$

$$x = 64.81 \text{ mg}$$

119. **The correct answer is (B).**

First simplify the numbers (see Answer 106); then use the law of exponents:

1. The product of two or more powers of the *same base* is the base with an exponent equal to the *sum of all the exponents*:

$$4^3 \times 4^{10} = 4^{10+3} = 4^{13}$$

2. The quotient of two powers with the *same base* is the base with an exponent equal to the *exponent of the numerator minus that of the denominator*:

$$\frac{3^8}{3^2} = 3^{8-2} = 3^6$$

3. The power of a power is found by *multiplying the exponents*:

$$(2^4)^3 = 2^{4 \times 3} = 2^{12}$$

4. The power of a product equals the *product of the powers* of the factors:

$$(2 \times 3 \times 4)^2 = 2^2 \times 3^2 \times 4^2$$

5. The root of a power is found by *dividing the exponent of the power by the index of the root*:

$$\sqrt[3]{8^6} = 8^{\frac{6}{3}} = 8^2$$

6. The power of a fraction equals the *power of the numerator divided by the power of the denominator*:

$$\left(\frac{2}{3}\right)^2 = \frac{2^2}{3^2}$$

7. A number with a *negative* exponent equals 1 divided by the number with a positive exponent:

$$12^{-2} = \frac{1}{12^2}$$

8. Any number other than 0 with exponent 0 equals 1:

$$10^0 = 1, \ 4^0 = 1, \ 1^0 = 1$$

Therefore, for Problem 119 we have $\sqrt[3]{3^6} = 3^{\frac{6}{3}} = 3^2$ and $\sqrt{2^2} = 2^{\frac{2}{2}} = 2^1 = 2$ so,

$$3^2 + 2 = (3 \times 3) + 2$$

$$3^2 + 2 = 11$$

120. **The correct answer is (A).**

Making the appropriate conversion to the least common denominator, we have

$$\left(\frac{2}{3}\right)^2 + 2^{-3} = \frac{2^2}{3^2} + \frac{1}{2^3}$$

$$= \frac{4}{9} + \frac{1}{8}$$

$$= \frac{4 \times 8}{9 \times 8} + \frac{9 \times 1}{9 \times 8}$$

$$= \frac{32}{72} + \frac{9}{72}$$

$$= \frac{41}{72}$$

121. **The correct answer is (C).**

$$10^0 = 1$$

$$10^1 = 10$$

$$\underline{10^{-1} = 0.1}$$

$$11.1$$

122.   The correct answer is (C).

In problems involving formulas, rearrange the formula until the unknown term is expressed by all the other terms. Therefore, if the temperature in degrees centigrade is unknown, rearrange the formula as follows:

$$9(x°C) = 5(y°F) - 160$$

$$x°C = \frac{5}{9}(y°F) - \frac{160}{9}$$

$$= \frac{5 \times 79}{9} - 17.78$$

$$= 26.1$$

123.   The correct answer is (B).

Rearrange to solve for the temperature in degrees Fahrenheit, as explained above:

$$9(x°C) = 5(y°F) - 160$$

$$5(x°F) = 9(x°C) + 160$$

$$x°F = \frac{9}{5}(x°C) + \frac{160}{5}$$

$$= \frac{9 \times (-10)}{5} + 32$$

$$= -18 + 32$$

$$= 14$$

124.   The correct answer is (D).

This problem may be approached by determining the respective temperatures in degrees centigrade and then computing the difference.

From

$$x°C = \frac{5(y°F) - 160}{9}$$

we have

$$x°C = \frac{5(72) - 160}{9}, \qquad x'°C = \frac{5(65) - 160}{9}$$

$$x°C = 22.22, \qquad\qquad x'°C \cong 18.33$$

So,

$$22.22 - 18.33 \cong 3.88 \qquad 3.9°C$$

Alternately, as one degree Fahrenheit is $\frac{9}{5}$ of a degree on the centigrade scale, the problem may be solved by multiplying the differences in degrees Fahrenheit by $\frac{5}{9}$.

$$72°F - 65°F = 7°F$$

$$7°F \times \frac{5}{9} = \frac{35}{9} = 3.88°C$$

You cannot directly substitute the 7°F into the temperature conversion equation as originally given, since that equation converts the 7°F to the corresponding temperature in degrees centigrade. That is, 7°F equals −13.8°C.

125.   The correct answer is (C).

This is a proportionality problem. Assume a weight-volume relationship

1:10,000::x:200:

$$\frac{1 \text{ g}}{10,000 \text{ ml}} = \frac{x \text{ g}}{200 \text{ ml}}$$

$$x \text{ g} = \frac{(1 \text{ g}) \times (200 \text{ ml})}{10,000 \text{ ml}}$$

$$= 0.02\text{g}$$

126.   The correct answer is (C).

When x is known, y may be found by drawing a line up from the x-axis, parallel to the y-axis, until the line of the graph is intersected. A line is then drawn from this point perpendicular to the y-axis until it is intersected. This is the value of y for a given x.

127.   The correct answer is (C).

The rate of drug disappearance is the change in y (mg drug/ml plasma) over a range of x (time). This is equal to the slope:

$$\frac{y_2 - y_1}{x_2 - x_1} = m$$

Therefore, to determine the rate (slope), any two y-values and corresponding x-values are needed: For example,

$$\text{time}_1 = 0 \text{ min}, \qquad y_1 = \frac{\text{mg drug}}{\text{ml plasma}} = 4$$

$$\text{time}_2 = 80 \text{ min}, \quad y_2 = \frac{\text{mg drug}}{\text{ml plasma}} = 2$$

Then,

$$\text{rate} = \frac{2-4}{80-0} = \frac{-2}{80} = \frac{-1}{40}$$

and

$$\frac{-1}{40} = \frac{-1\text{mg}/\text{ml plasma}}{40 \text{ min}} = -1.5 \text{ mg/ml plasma per hour}$$

Note: The negative sign indicates a decline, or falling y values, for increasing x values.

128. The correct answer is (B).

To predict a y value for a given x, the slope m and the y-intercept b must be known so we can solve $y - mx + b$. From Answer 127,

$$m = \frac{-1.5 \text{ mg / ml plasma}}{1 \text{ hr.}}$$

and

$$b = 4 \text{ mg/ml plasma}$$

$$x = 2 \text{ hr}$$

So,

$$y = (-1.5 \text{ mg/ml per hour}) \times (2 \text{ hr}) + 4 \text{ mg/ml}$$

$$= -3.0 \text{ mg/ml} + 4 \text{ mg/ml}$$

$$= 1.0 \text{ mg/ml}$$

Remember to include the negative sign in the slope.

129. The correct answer is (A).

In this problem, the y-intercept has been changed to 8 mg/ml and the time to 80 min (1.33 hr). The problem is then solved as above:

$$y = mx + b$$

$$= (-1.5 \text{ mg/ml per hour [ts] } (1.33 \text{ hr}) + 8 \text{ mg/hr}$$

$$= -1.995 + 8$$

$$\cong 6 \text{ mg/ml}$$

130. The correct answer is (C).

This problem requires finding the value of x (time) when y (concentration) is zero. Again,

$$y \text{ is } mx + b$$

$$0 = (-1.5 \text{ mg/ml per hour})x + 4 \text{ mg/ml}$$

$$\frac{-4 \text{ mg / ml}}{-1.5 \text{ mg / ml per hour}} = x$$

$$2.66 \text{ hr} = x$$

$$160 \text{ min} = x$$

131. The correct answer is (C).

An integer is any of the natural numbers, the negatives of the numbers and zero. To find the values for the inequalities, solve each of the inequalities separately; then delete all values *not* satisfying *both*:

$4 < 3x - 2 \leq 10$	$3x - 2 \leq 10$
$4 < 3x - 2$	$3x \leq 10 + 2$
$4 + 2 < 3x$	$3x \leq 12$
$\dfrac{6}{3} < x$	$x \leq 4$
$2 < x$	

Therefore, all values greater than 2 may be accepted: $3, 4, 5, ..., n$

Therefore, all values less than or equal to 4 will be accepted: $4, 3, 2, 1, 0, -1, -2, ..., -n$

Integer values common to both inequalities are 3 and 4.

132. **The correct answer is (B).**

$$\frac{7}{x} > 2, \quad x \neq 0$$

$$7 > 2x$$

$$\frac{7}{2} > x$$

$$3.5 > x$$

x must be less than 3.5, or 3, 2, 1, 0, -1, -2..., but x cannot be 0; therefore 3, 2, 1 are common to both equations.

133. **The correct answer is (C).**

The absolute value $|x|$ removes the sign of the number enclosed after all arithmetic functions enclosed have been completed, or $|-x| = x$.

Therefore

$$|-5| - |-2| = 5 - 2 = 3$$

134. **The correct answer is (A).**

$$|8 - 14| = |-6| = 6$$

135. **The correct answer is (D).**

$$|5x + 4| = -3$$

This problem cannot be solved, as there is no term whose absolute value will yield a negative result.

136. **The correct answer is (B).**

As the figure is a cube, D is the hypotenuse of a right triangle with equal sides. From the Pythagorean Theorem, we have hypotenuse^2 = side^2 + side^2

$$x^2 = 2^2 + 2^2$$

$$x^2 = 4 + 4$$

$$x^2 = 8$$

$$x = \sqrt{8}$$

137. **The correct answer is (A).**

In this example, lines C, D, and E form a right triangle with base D and side C (or base C and side D). If C is 2 in. (given condition) and D, from the previous example, is $\sqrt{8}$ in., then $\frac{1}{2}\sqrt{8}(2) = \sqrt{8}$ in.^{2} (The area of a triangle is equal to $\frac{1}{2}$ base $\times$ height.) E could also serve as a base, except, as E was unknown, it was easier to work with the sides already known.

138. **The correct answer is (A).**

A cube has six faces: top, bottom, and four sides. If each face has a surface area of 2×2 in.^{2}, then the total area is

$$\frac{(2 \text{ in.} \times 2 \text{ in.})}{\text{face} \times 6 \text{ faces}} = 24 \text{ in.}^2$$

139. **The correct answer is (D).**

The subset of $\underline{A \text{ or } B}$ includes all subsets for A (1, 2) plus all subsets of B (2, 3, 4); that is, all cases in which the condition of $\underline{A \text{ or } B}$ has been met will be accepted (1, 2, 3, 4).

140. **The correct answer is (B).**

A subset $\underline{A \text{ and } B}$ includes all cases in which *both* the conditions of subset A and subset B must be met (2 only).

141. **The correct answer is (A).**

The subset $\underline{A \text{ or } C}$ includes all cases satisfying the conditions of subset A (1, 2) plus those satisfying the conditions of C (4, 5). However, any cases also included in B must be excluded (2, 3, or 4), for the subset we are looking for is $\underline{A \text{ or } C, \text{ but not } B}$. Therefore, only subsets 1 and 5 may be accepted.

142. **The correct answer is (D).**

The subset "only" means that any other conditions being met must be excluded. Therefore, although B is composed of 2, 3, and 4, only 3 may be accepted, as 2 is also a subset of A and 4 is also a subset of C.

143. **The correct answer is (B).**

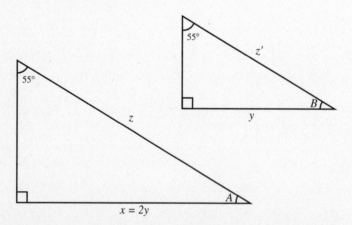

The ratio of the areas of similar triangles is equal to the square of the ratio of corresponding sides. Therefore, when $x = 2y$, the ratio of the sides is $\frac{2}{1} : \frac{x}{y}$ as x is twice the value of y. The ratio of the areas is then $\left(\frac{2}{1}\right)^2$ or $\frac{4}{1}$ or 4:1.

144.   The correct answer is (D).

The sum of all angles in a triangle is 180°. If one angle is 55° and a right angle is 90°, then angle *A* is 180° – 55° – 90° = 35°.

145.   The correct answer is (D).

Since the two triangles are similar, if $x = 3y$, then

$$z = 3\,z', \text{ or}$$

$$z' = \frac{z}{3} = \frac{5}{3} = 1\frac{2}{3}$$

146.   The correct answer is (B).

The value of a bar graph is determined by drawing a line perpendicular to the *y* axis from the top of the graph. The point of interception is the *y*-value of that bar.

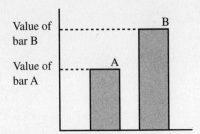

Therefore, only B and C have 90% or more of the active ingredient as declared by the manufacturer.

147.   The correct answer is (C).

If sample B was 100% of claim and C was 120%, then the amount of drug present is

$$100\% \times 200 \text{ mg} = 1 \times 200 = 200 \text{ mg}$$

$$120\% \times 200 \text{ mg} = 1.2 \times 200 = 240 \text{ mg}$$

148.   The correct answer is (C).

The mean is the sum of all values divided by the number of samples:

$$\overline{X} = \frac{1}{N} \Sigma\, x \text{ when } N \text{ is the number of samples and } x \text{ is the value of each sample. From the bar graph, the}$$

following values were obtained:

1 score of 20	20 = (1 × 20)	5 scores of 70	350 = (5 × 70)
1 score of 30	30 = (1 × 30)	4 scores of 80	320 = (4 × 80)
1 score of 40	40 = (1 × 40)	2 scores of 90	180 = (2 × 90)
2 scores of 50	100 = (2 × 50)	1 score of 100	100 = (1 × 100)
3 scores of 60	180 = (3 × 60)		

N = 20 = number of samples   Σ of all values = 1320

$$\frac{1}{N} \Sigma\, x = \frac{1320}{20} = 66.0 = \text{mean}$$

149.   The correct answer is (A).

The modal score is the most frequently occurring score. As five students scored 70% and no other score occurred as frequently, 70% is the modal score.

150.   The correct answer is (A).

The median is the term that is larger than or equal to half the terms and equal to or smaller than the other half of them. In this example, there are scores for a total of 20 students. As there are an even number of terms, there exists no actual median; that is, no term larger than exactly half of the terms and smaller than the other half. But now it is possible to find two middle terms, and the median is defined as the mean of these two middle terms. In this example, if the scores are ranked in ascending order, the two middle scores are 70 and 70:

1.	20	6.	60	*11.	70	16.	80
2.	30	7.	60	12.	70	17.	80
3.	40	8.	60	13.	70	18.	90
4.	50	9.	70	14.	80	19.	90
5.	50	*10.	70	15.	80	20.	100

*As rank position, 10 and 11 are in the middle; that is, 70 is larger than or equal to half of the terms and equal to or smaller than half, and as 70 is the mean of 70 and 70, the median is 70.

151.   The correct answer is (A).

This is a proportionality problem:

$$0.625 \text{ g}:50::31.25 \text{ g}:x$$

$$\frac{0.625}{2050} = \frac{31.25}{x}$$

$$x \text{ tablets} = \frac{31.25 \text{ g} \times 50 \text{ tablets}}{0.625 \text{ g}}$$

$$= 2,500 \text{ tablets}$$

152.   The correct answer is (B).

Assuming that the dose should be directly related to body weight, we set up a proportion:

$$\frac{70 \ \mu g}{150 \text{ lb}} = \frac{x \ \mu g}{44 \text{ lb}}$$

$$x \mu g = \frac{70 \ \mu g \times 44 \text{ lb}}{150 \text{ lb}}$$

$$x = 20.53 \ \mu g \cong 20 \ \mu g$$

153. **The correct answer is (B).**

To solve for changes in y relative to x, rearrange the equation in terms of y:

$$x = \frac{1}{y}$$

$$y = \frac{1}{x}$$

Then substitute in the change:

$$y = \frac{1}{x(2)} = \left(\frac{1}{x}\right) \times \frac{1}{2}$$

Therefore, it can be seen that when x increases by a factor of 2, y is halved.

154. **The correct answer is (A).**

Rearrange the equation in terms of y (see above):

$$x = 2y$$

$$y = \frac{x}{2}$$

Increase x by a factor of 2:

$$y = \frac{x \times 2}{2}$$

y has increased by a factor of 2.

155. **The correct answer is (D).**

This is a simple fraction problem. The question is, How many times does 16 go into 24?

$$\frac{24 \text{ g}}{16} = 1.5 \text{ g} = 1,500 \text{ mg}$$

156. **The correct answer is (D).**

Determine the weight that represents a 10% error. The range of acceptable weights would be all the tablet weights that are within 150 g ± the 10% error:

$$150 \text{ g} \times \frac{10\%}{100\%} = 15 \text{ g}$$

$$150 \text{ g} - 15 \text{ g} = 135 \text{ g}$$

$$150 \text{ g} + 15 \text{ g} = 165 \text{ g}$$

So, the range is 135–165 g.

157. The correct answer is (A).

A percentage is the amount per hundred. A proportion should then be set up to find how much iron is in 100 mg of ferrous sulfate, knowing the ratio of 65 mg/325 mg, iron to ferrous sulfate:

$$\frac{x}{100\%} = \frac{65 \text{ mg of iron}}{325 \text{ mg of ferrous sulfate}}$$

$$\frac{65 \text{ mg}}{325 \text{ mg}} \times 100\% = 20\%$$

158. The correct answer is (D).

Set up a proportion with x representing the number of milligrams of compound in a liter (remember, 1 liter equals 1,000 ml):

$$\frac{x \text{ mg}}{1,000 \text{ ml}} = \frac{50 \text{ mg}}{\text{ml}}$$

$$x \text{ mg} = \frac{50 \text{ mg} \times 1,000 \text{ ml}}{\text{ml}}$$

$$= 50,000 \text{ mg}$$

As 1,000 mg are in 1 g,

$$\frac{50,000 \text{ g}}{1,000 \text{ mg} / 1 \text{ g}} = 50 \text{ g}$$

159. The correct answer is (B).

If 5 ml is the smallest unit marked, then all errors are related to this unit and all readings would be rounded off to multiples of that unit; 5 ml represents the potential error. In this problem, the potential error is also the percentage error of a measured volume (x ml):

$$\frac{5 \text{ ml}}{x \text{ ml}} \times 100\% = \text{percentage error}$$

$$\frac{500\%}{x \text{ ml}} = 10\%$$

$$x \text{ ml} = \frac{500\%}{10\%}$$

$$x = 50 \text{ ml}$$

160. The correct answer is (B).

The average is analogous to the mean:

$$\frac{1}{N} \Sigma \text{ values} = \text{average}$$

$$\frac{61 + 50 + 100 + 50}{1 + 1 + 1 + 1} = 65.25 = 65$$

161. **The correct answer is (C).**

The equation for a straight line is $y = mx + b$, where b is the y intercept and m is the slope.

Thus,

$$y = mx + b$$

$$y = -0.118x + 8.5$$

162. **The correct answer is (A).**

Rearrange the equation of the line to isolate x; then, substitute the value of the y-intercept:

$$y = -0.118x + 8.5$$

$$y - 8.5 = -0.118x$$

$$\left[\frac{y - 8.5}{-0.118}\right] = x$$

$$\left[\frac{6 - 8.5}{-0.118}\right] = x$$

$$21 = x$$

163. **The correct answer is (C).**

The value of y, when x is zero, is the y-intercept (8.5). For all other values of x, solve for y by substituting into the equation of the line.

164. **The correct answer is (C).**

The volume of the cylinder is $\pi r^2 h$, where h (height) is 10 and r (radius) is 2:

$$\text{volume} = \pi r^2 h$$

$$= (3.14)(2^2)(10)$$

$$= 125.6 \text{ units}^3$$

$$= 126 \text{ units}^3$$

165. **The correct answer is (C).**

The lateral surface area is the circumference of the end, $2\pi r$, times the height:

$$\text{Lateral surface} = (2\pi r)(h)$$

$$= (2)(3.14)(2)(10)$$

$$= 125.6$$

$$= 126 \text{ units}^2$$

166. **The correct answer is (B).**

The total area is the area of the lateral surface plus the areas of both ends:

area of circle $= \pi r^2$

lateral surface $= 2\pi rh$

total area $= (2)(\pi r^2) + (2\pi rh)$

$\qquad = 2\pi r\,(r + h)$

$\qquad = (2)\,(3.14)\,(2)\,(2 + 10)$

$\qquad = 150.7$

167. **The correct answer is (B).**

The area of a trapezoid is $\frac{1}{2}(h)\,(a + b)$:

$$\frac{1}{2}(1)\,(4 + 2) = \text{area}$$

$$3 \text{ units}^2 = \text{area}$$

168. **The correct answer is (C).**

The area of a parallelogram is determined by $h \times b$:

$$(2)(5) = \text{area}$$

$$10 \text{ units}^2 = \text{area}$$

169. **The correct answer is (C).**

To solve simultaneous equations, isolate the term in the first equation, which will be subsequently inserted into the second equation. In this case, y will be expressed in terms of x and b. The a term is common to both; therefore, rearrange the x equation to isolate a:

$x = 3b + a$

$a = x - 3b$

Then, substitute into the y equation:

$y = 3a + b = 3(x - 3b) + b$

$\qquad = 3x - 9b + b = 3x - 8b$

170. **The correct answer is (A).**

The slope of a line (m) is the change in y versus the change in x (x versus y). Therefore, the correct answer is (A), a slope of m. The ordinate (y-value) intercept is given by c. The abscissa (x-value) intercept occurs when y equals zero or $0 = m\,x + c$, $x = \dfrac{-c}{m}$.

171. The correct answer is (D).

When one divides ratios with the same denominator, the denominators may be factored out and only the numerators divided. It may be viewed in any of the following fashions:

$$\frac{7 \div 3}{21 \div 3} = \frac{7}{21} = \frac{1}{3} = 0.33$$

$$7:3::21:3 \rightarrow \frac{7}{21} = \frac{1}{3} = 0.33$$

$$\frac{7}{3} \div \frac{21}{3} = \frac{7}{21} = \frac{1}{3} = 0.33$$

172. The correct answer is (D).

To reduce a fraction, first determine what roots of the numerator are common in the denominator:

$$\frac{72}{2,880} = \frac{72}{72 \times 40} \text{ or } \frac{2 \times 2 \times 2 \times 3 \times 3}{2 \times 2 \times 2 \times 2 \times 2 \times 2 \times 3 \times 3 \times 5}$$

$$= \frac{1}{2 \times 2 \times 2 \times 5}$$

$$= \frac{1}{40}$$

173. The correct answer is (A).

Set up the proportion:

$$\frac{0.25 \text{ mg}}{\text{tablet}} = \frac{7.5 \text{ mg}}{x \text{ tablets}}$$

$$x = \frac{7.5 \text{ mg} \times 1 \text{ tablet}}{0.25 \text{ mg}}$$

$$x = 30$$

174. The correct answer is (C).

Convert all the fractions to decimals; then, add all values:

$$\frac{3}{4} = \frac{x}{1.00} \qquad \frac{2}{5} = \frac{x}{1.00}$$

$$x = \frac{3 \times 1.00}{4} \qquad x = \frac{2 \times 1.00}{5}$$

$$x = 0.75 \qquad x = 0.40$$

$$\frac{3}{4} \text{ mg} + 0.25 \text{ mg} + \frac{2}{5} \text{ mg} + 2.75 \text{ mg} = x \text{ mg}$$

$$0.75 + 0.25 + 0.40 + 2.75 = 4.15 \text{ mg}$$

175. The correct answer is (A).

To add, convert all numbers to common units. In this case, grams (g) is the base unit:

$$1,000 \text{ mg} = 1 \text{ g}$$

$$1 \text{ kg} = 1,000 \text{ g}$$

Therefore,

$$\frac{0.75 \text{ mg}}{x \text{ g}} = \frac{1,000 \text{ mg}}{1 \text{ g}}$$

$$x \text{ g} = 0.00075 \text{ g}$$

$$\frac{0.5 \text{ kg}}{x \text{ g}} = \frac{1 \text{ kg}}{1,000 \text{ g}}$$

$$x \text{ g} = 500 \text{ g}$$

$$0.75 \text{ mg} + 50 \text{ g} + 0.5 \text{ kg} - x \text{ g}$$

$$0.00075 \text{ g} + 50 \text{ g} + 500 \text{ g} = 550.00075 \text{ g}$$

176. The correct answer is (B).

Express $3\frac{1}{8}$ as a fraction:

$$\frac{3 \times 8}{8} + \frac{1}{8} = \frac{25}{8}$$

Then, convert the fraction so that it has a denominator common to those of the possible answers. Those values with a denominator of 36 may automatically be discarded, as 8 is not a factor of 36, (i.e., 36 cannot be divided by 8 to yield a whole number). Therefore, only denominators of 32 need be considered:

$$\frac{25 \times 4}{8 \times 4} = \frac{100}{32}$$

177. The correct answer is (B).

First determine how many milligrams are being considered; then convert to grains by proportionalities:

$$\frac{10\%}{100\%} \times 360 = 36 \text{ mg}$$

$$\frac{1 \text{ g}}{60 \text{ mg}} = \frac{x \text{ g}}{36 \text{ mg}}$$

$$x \text{ grains} = 0.6 \text{ grain}$$

178. The correct answer is (D).

Both quantities must first be converted to similar denominators; then they can be simplified and added:

$$\frac{2\sqrt{36} \times 3\sqrt{7}}{3\sqrt{7}} + \frac{4\sqrt{28}}{3\sqrt{7}} = \frac{\left(2\sqrt{6 \times 6} \times 3\sqrt{7}\right)}{3\sqrt{7}} + \frac{4\sqrt{2 \times 2 \times 7}}{3\sqrt{7}}$$

$$= \frac{(2 \times 6) \times \left(3\sqrt{7}\right) + 4\sqrt{2 \times 2} \times \sqrt{7}}{3\sqrt{7}}$$

$$= \frac{36 + 8}{3}$$

$$= 14\frac{2}{3}$$

179. The correct answer is (A).

This is a simple subtraction problem. If A were equal to x, then $1 + A$ would equal $1 + x$. The value of A does not change the mathematical principle. Therefore, when

$$A = e^a$$

we have

$$1 + A = 1 + e^a$$

180. The correct answer is (C).

Any number to the power of zero is 1:

$$7.7 \times 10^0 = 7.7 \times 1 = 7.7$$

181. The correct answer is (C).

1,000,000 expressed in base 10 is 1×10^6. Using the law of exponents (see Answer 119), we have

$$1 \times 10^3 \times 10^3 = 1 \times 10^{3+3}$$

$$= 1 \times 10^6$$

182. The correct answer is (D).

Using the law of exponents (see Answer 119), we see that $\sqrt{144 \times 10^4}$ may be broken down as follows:

$$\sqrt{144 \times 10^4} = \sqrt{144} \times \sqrt{10^4}$$

$$= \sqrt{12 \times 12} \times \sqrt{10^2 \times 10^2}$$

$$= 12 \times 10^2$$

$$= 1,200$$

183. **The correct answer is (A).**

Using proportionalities to convert the total weight after summing, we have 132 lbs + 11 lbs + 44 lbs = 187 lbs. So, then

$$\frac{1 \text{ kg}}{2.2 \text{ lbs}} = \frac{x \text{ kg}}{187 \text{ lbs}}$$

$$\frac{1 \text{ kg} \times 187 \text{ lbs}}{2.2 \text{ lbs}} = x \text{ kg}$$

$$x \text{ kg} = 85 \text{ kg}$$

184. **The correct answer is (B).**

Simply convert to a common denominator and add (see Answer 119):

$$\left(\frac{3}{4}\right)^2 = \frac{3^2}{4^2} = \frac{9}{14}$$

$$3^2 = 9$$

$$\sqrt{\frac{49}{256}} = \frac{\sqrt{49}}{\sqrt{256}} = \frac{\sqrt{7 \times 7}}{\sqrt{2 \times 2 \times 2 \times 2 \times 2 \times 2 \times 2 \times 2}}$$

$$= \frac{7}{\sqrt{2^8}} = \frac{7}{\sqrt{2^4}} = \frac{7}{16}$$

Therefore,

$$\frac{3^2}{4} + 3^2 + \sqrt{\frac{49}{256}} = x$$

$$\frac{9}{16} + \frac{9 \times 16}{16} + \frac{7}{16} = x$$

$$x = \frac{160}{16} = 10$$

185. **The correct answer is (C).**

The equation of a line is $y = mx + b$ (see Answers 126 – 128), where m is the slope and b is the y-intercept. Therefore,

$$y = mx + b$$

$$y = -2x + \sqrt{2}$$

186. **The correct answer is (D).**

Simplify the numerator; then, divide the result by the denominator:

$$250,000 \times 0.018 = 4500.000. = 4,500$$

$$\frac{4,500}{0.15} = 30000.00$$

$$= 30,000$$

187.   The correct answer is (A).

If we use the law of exponents, $x^{-3} = \dfrac{1}{x^3}$, then

$$\dfrac{1}{x^3} = \dfrac{1}{27}$$

$$x^3 = 27$$

$$x = \sqrt[3]{27} = \sqrt[3]{3 \times 3 \times 3}$$

$$= 3$$

188.   The correct answer is (A).

Corresponding sides of similar triangles are related by the same ratio. Therefore,

$$\dfrac{J}{K} = \text{ratio of one side}$$

$$\dfrac{H}{I} = \text{ratio of second side}$$

$$\dfrac{J}{K} = \dfrac{H}{I}$$

$$I = \dfrac{KH}{J}$$

189.   The correct answer is (A).

If drug A is 20% of the compound, then drug A is 20% of 500 g.

$$\dfrac{20\%}{100\%} \times 500 = \text{grams of drug A}$$

$$\dfrac{10,000}{100} = \text{grams of drug A} = 100$$

190.   The correct answer is (B).

Drugs A and B represent 20 and 5%, respectively, of the compound. Therefore, 25% of 500 g is the amount of drugs A and B.

$$\dfrac{20}{100} + \dfrac{5}{100} \times 500 \text{ g} = \text{grams of drugs A and B}$$

$$\dfrac{12,500}{100} = \text{grams of drugs A and B} = 125 \text{ g}$$

191. The correct answer is (D).

Drugs B and C represent 5% and 75%, respectively, of the compound. Therefore, 80% of 500 g is the amount of drugs B and C.

$$\frac{5}{100} + \frac{75}{100} \times 500 \text{ g} = \text{grams of drugs B and C}$$

$$\frac{40,000}{100} = \text{grams of drugs B and C} = 400$$

192. The correct answer is (A).

Drugs A, B, and C represent 20%, 5%, and 75% of the compound, which, when summed, make up 100% of the compound. Therefore, 100 g of drugs A, B, and C are in 100 g of the compound.

193. The correct answer is (B).

The ratios A:B:C are 20%:5%:75%.

If 5 is the lowest common denominator, then

$$\frac{20}{5} : \frac{5}{5} : \frac{75}{5}$$

4:1:15

194. The correct answer is (D).

If this problem is approached as a proportion, then the product of the means divided by one of the extremes equals the other extreme. Initially, isolate the extreme $g_b M_b$:

$$\frac{B-p}{q} = \frac{g_b M_a}{g_b M_b}$$

$$g_b M_b = \frac{(g_a M_a)(q)}{B-p}$$

Again, treat the equation as a proportion and isolate the extreme (g_b):

$$g_b = \frac{(g_a M_a)(q)(M_b)}{B-p}$$

that upon rearrangement, yields

$$g_b = \left[\frac{q}{B-p}\right]\left[\frac{M_b(g_a)}{M_a}\right]$$

195. The correct answer is (D).

From the equation for a straight line (see Answers 126–128), $y = mx + b$:

	y-intercept (b)	slope (m)	x-intercept ($y = 0$)
Equation 1	4	+3	−4/3
Equation 2	−4	+3	4/3

196. The correct answer is (A).

To solve simultaneous equations, express the first equation in terms of a single unknown term (I). Then substitute this value into the second equation and solve for the second unknown (II). After solving for the second unknown, substitute its value back into the first equation and solve for the remaining unknown term (III):

$$30 = a + 3b - 70 \qquad\qquad \text{(I)}$$

$$a = 30 - 3b + 70$$

$$3a + 5b = 100 \qquad\qquad \text{(II)}$$

$$3(30 - 3b + 70) + 5b = 100$$

$$90 - 9b + 210 + 5b = 100$$

$$-4b = 100 - 210 - 90$$

$$4b = 200$$

$$b = 50$$

$$30 = a + 3b - 70 \qquad\qquad \text{(III)}$$

$$30 = a + 3(50) - 70$$

$$30 = a + 150 - 70$$

$$a = -50$$

197. The correct answer is (B).

The question is really asking what is the total volume used. This is the total volume of a dose times the number of doses, which is then expressed in milliliters:

$$\frac{2 \text{ tablespoonfuls}}{\text{dose}} \times \frac{2 \text{ doses}}{\text{day}} \times 10 \text{ days} = \text{total volume}$$

$$40 \text{ tablespoonfuls} \times \frac{15 \text{ ml}}{\text{tablespoonful}} = 600 \text{ ml}$$

198.   The correct answer is (D).

This problem is solved with proportions; however, as we will be dividing the total weight into smaller units, the weight should be converted to a smaller unit to minimize the number of decimal places of which we will have to keep track:

$$0.060 \text{ g} \times \frac{1,000 \text{ mg}}{1 \text{ g}} = 60 \text{ mg}$$

$$\frac{60 \text{ mg}}{125 \text{ tablets}} = \frac{x \text{ mg}}{\text{tablet}}$$

$$0.480 \text{ mg} = \frac{x \text{ mg}}{\text{tablet}}$$

$$0.480 \text{ mg} \times \frac{1,000 \text{ g}}{\text{mg}} = 480 \text{ g}$$

199.   The correct answer is (C).

This is a conversion problem, which again is easiest to solve by the use of proportions:

$$\frac{1 \text{ in.}}{2.54 \text{ cm.}} = \frac{x \text{ in.}}{12.70 \text{ cm.}}$$

$$\frac{12.70 \times 1 \text{ in.}}{2.54 \text{ cm.}} = x \text{ in.}$$

$$5 \text{ in.} = x$$

200.   The correct answer is (A).

To divide fractions, invert the second term and multiply:

$$\frac{1}{120} \div \frac{1}{150} = \frac{1}{120} \times \frac{150}{1} = \frac{150}{120}$$

Then simplify and complete the multiplication:

$$\frac{150}{120} = \frac{15}{12} = \frac{5 \times 3}{4 \times 3} = \frac{5}{4}$$

$$\frac{5}{4} \times 50 = \frac{250}{4} = 62\frac{1}{2}$$

Explanatory Answers
Test 3: Biology

201. **The correct answer is (C).**

The cell is the smallest unit of life that can survive independently. The gene of a cell resides in the nucleus of the cell and can be considered an organelle, or part of the cellular machinery. An organ is composed of living cells.

202. **The correct answer is (B).**

The mitochondria is the primary source of energy for the aerobic cell. The endoplasmic reticulum and Golgi apparatus use energy from the mitochondria to synthesize and store cellular products. The nucleus is primarily responsible for the storage of genetic information.

203. **The correct answer is (B).**

By using a Punnett square, we see that two *Bb* individuals have a 1-in-4 (25%) chance of producing an offspring with blue (bb) eyes.

	B	*b*
B	*BB*	*Bb*
b	Bb	bb

204. **The correct answer is (C).**

Hypertonic solutions have a greater salt, or electrolyte, concentration than do red blood cells. Therefore, water leaves blood cells and enters the hypertonic solution, causing the red blood cells to shrink. Both isotonic and iso-osmotic solutions will have no effect on the red blood cells. A hypotonic solution will cause water to enter the red blood cells because of their higher electrolyte concentration and cause the cells to swell.

205. **The correct answer is (D).**

Copper is considered a trace element that is necessary for normal metabolism of the body. Sodium, potassium, and calcium are major elements vital to the healthy body.

206. **The correct answer is (D).**

	B	*B*
b	*Bb*	*Bb*
b	Bb	Bb

A cross between a homozygous brown individual (*BB*) and a homozygous white individual (*bb*) will result in all offspring being brown heterozygous (*Bb*), as seen in the Punnett square.

207. The correct answer is (B).

Vitamins A, D, E, and K are fat-soluble vitamins. All the B vitamins, as well as vitamin C, are water-soluble vitamins.

208. The correct answer is (A).

Under basal conditions, the liver receives about 25% of the total cardiac output, whereas the brain and skeletal muscle receive about 15%. The bone is relatively nonvascularized and receives only 5% of the total blood flow.

209. The correct answer is (A).

Sodium is the most abundant electrolyte in extracellular fluid (~142 mEq/liter) with potassium the most abundant electrolyte (~141 mEq/liter) inside the cell (intracellular fluid). Both calcium (0–5 mEq/liter) and magnesium (3–58 mEq/liter) exist in relatively small amounts in the extracellular fluid.

210. The correct answer is (C).

The small intestine has the largest surface area and carries out most of the specialized transport mechanisms in the gastrointestinal tract. Very little absorption of nutrients occurs in the stomach or the large intestine, also referred to as the colon.

211. The correct answer is (D).

Long-chain (more than 10 carbons) fatty acids normally enter the circulatory system by way of the lymphatic system, packaged as chylomicrons. Short-chain fatty acids normally enter the circulatory system directly as free fatty acids.

212. The correct answer is (B).

See the explanation for Answer 209.

213. The correct answer is (A).

Scurvy is a disease resulting from a vitamin C deficiency. Deficiencies in thiamine, niacin, and vitamin D result in beriberi, pellagra, and rickets, respectively.

214. The correct answer is (C).

Squamous epithelium is normally associated with body surfaces, as a form of protection (i.e., skin). Epithelium associated with the kidney, lungs, and pancreas is more suited for secretory functions and is columnar or cuboidal in nature.

215. The correct answer is (B).

Chromatin is composed of DNA and protein and is found primarily in the nucleus.

216. The correct answer is (A).

Skeletal muscle fibers contract and relax in about 0.1 second. Cardiac muscle requires 1–5 seconds, whereas smooth muscle needs more than 3 seconds to contract and relax.

217. The correct answer is (B).

Saturated fats have all their carbon bonds saturated with hydrogens; thus, there are no double bonds. As the number of double bonds increases, the melting point of the fat decreases. Therefore, saturated fats are normally solids at room temperature, whereas unsaturated fats are liquids. Complete oxidation of 1 g of fat yields about 9 calories, whereas 1 g of carbohydrate yields about 4 calories.

218. The correct answer is (C).

Messenger RNA transfers genetic information from the nucleus by forming a complex with the ribosomes (composed largely of ribosomal RNA) of the endoplasmic reticulum in the cytoplasm. Transfer RNA carries amino acids to the messenger RNA-ribosome complex during protein synthesis.

219. The correct answer is (D).

Each mitotic division is a continuous process, with each stage merging imperceptibly into the next. For descriptive purposes, mitosis is divided into four successive stages: prophase, metaphase, anaphase, and telophase.

220. The correct answer is (B).

Since biological membranes are primarily a sandwich composed of a bimolecular layer of lipid with a layer of protein on both the inner and outer surfaces, lipid-soluble compounds diffuse through it faster than water-soluble compounds. For water-soluble compounds, the size of the molecule is the rate-limiting factor in diffusion.

221. The correct answer is (D).

Passive diffusion of a substance requires no energy (ATP) and will therefore not be affected by a metabolic inhibitor (cyanide). Passive diffusion also transfers uncharged (more lipid-soluble) molecules from a higher to a lower concentration.

222. The correct answer is (A).

A large sodium (Na^+) influx into the cell results in the resting potential (–50 mV) becoming more positive and thereby initiates the action potential. Potassium is already in very high concentration (~141 mEq/liter) intracellularly and will not enter the cell.

223. The correct answer is (D).

A large efflux of potassium (K^+) out of the cell results in a fall in electrical potential within the cell. Potassium, in high concentration intracellularly, easily leaves the cell, whereas sodium, in high concentration extracellularly, will not diffuse out of the cell rapidly.

224. The correct answer is (C).

The normal resting potential of –50 mV is established by the sodium-potassium pump of the cell, resulting in a high extracellular sodium concentration (~142 mEq/liter) and a high intracellular potassium concentration (A~141 mE~/liter). A negative resting potential is necessary to allow proper initiation of an action potential.

225. **The correct answer is (B).**

Insulin is a hormone that decreases blood glucose levels by increasing glucose uptake and storage by the cells. Pepsin, trypsin, and lactase are enzymes necessary for the proper digestion of nutrients.

226. **The correct answer is (C).**

The liver is the primary site of metabolism for the body and is responsible for detoxifying toxic agents in the blood. The lungs and kidneys both excrete these metabolized agents from the body. The pancreas does not directly metabolize toxic agents to any extent.

227. **The correct answer is (C).**

The kidneys remove waste products from the body.

228. **The correct answer is (D).**

All these processes are involved in the absorption of carbohydrates, amino acids, and fatty acids, as well as minerals and vitamins.

229. **The correct answer is (A).**

Bile salts are necessary for the proper digestion of fats in that they emulsify fat globules and render the end products of fat digestion soluble for more efficient absorption.

230. **The correct answer is (C).**

Glucose, fructose, and galactose are all simple sugars derived from hydrolytic cleavage of polysaccharides and double sugars. These simple sugars are then readily absorbed from the digestive tract. Glycogen is the storage form of glucose in the different cells of the body.

231. **The correct answer is (A).**

The brain does not store glucose as glycogen and must receive all its energy from glucose in the blood. Therefore, a rapid decrease in blood glucose immediately deprives the brain of the energy source it requires for normal function.

232. **The correct answer is (D).**

Vitamin A, or retinol, is converted in the retina to retinal, a light-sensitive pigment, necessary for night vision.

233. **The correct answer is (B).**

Both active transport and facilitated diffusion require carriers that combine with the transported substance. Passive diffusion involves the transfer of a substance from a region of higher concentration to one of lower concentration without a carrier.

234. **The correct answer is (B).**

Saturation of the carrier with the transferring substance in active transport and facilitated diffusion will lead to saturation kinetics. In addition, phagocytosis also has a maximum rate of transfer. Passive diffusion does not have any of these restrictions and normally proceeds at a rate proportional to the amount of substance present for transfer.

235. The correct answer is (C).

Mendel's first law, called the law of segregation, states that genes exist in individuals as pairs. The theory of recapitulation states that organisms tend to repeat, in the course of their evolutionary development, some of the corresponding stages of their evolutionary ancestors. Starling's law, also known as Starling's law of the heart, deals with regulation of the amount of blood pumped by the heart at a given time. The Watson-Crick model explains how the DNA molecule transfers information and undergoes replication.

236. The correct answer is (D).

About 56% of the adult human body is water (H_2O), with the rest of the body being primarily composed of organic molecules containing carbon. Therefore, of the four stated elements, calcium would be the least abundant in the human body.

237. The correct answer is (C).

Most species of animals and plants have chromosome numbers between 10 and 50. Humans have 46 chromosomes in each of their cells. Abnormalities in the chromosome number include Turner's syndrome (45 chromosomes) and Klinefelter's syndrome (47 chromosomes).

238. The correct answer is (A).

O-negative blood, by definition, contains no A, B, or Rh agglutinogens that would cause a transfusion reaction and possibly death for a blood recipient. Therefore, O-negative blood can be given to any individuals of the four major blood types.

239. The correct answer is (D).

Epinephrine is one of the neurotransmitters in the brain, especially in the thalamus and hypothalamus. Both norepinephrine and acetylcholine are transmitter substances known to be secreted by the autonomic nerves innervating smooth muscle. Cholecystokinin is a hormone secreted by the intestinal mucosa that causes specific contraction of the gallbladder.

240. The correct answer is (D).

Neutrophils, monocytes, eosinophils, and basophils are white blood cells produced by the bone marrow along with red blood cells. Lymphocytes are white blood cells that are produced by lymphoid tissue.

241. The correct answer is (A).

Actively acquired immunity depends upon the production of specific proteins, antibodies, that are released into the blood and tissue fluids in response to some foreign protein (an antigen) or vaccine. On the other hand, passively acquired immunity is a result of the injection of antibodies that have been produced in another individual or species. Natural immunity protects humans from infectious diseases associated with animals, such as canine distemper. Cellular immunity deals with the recognition and destruction of foreign, genetically different cells, and may be the cause of the rejection of transplanted organs.

242. The correct answer is (C).

Glomerular filtration is the process by which the kidney removes most of the waste products from the blood by pure filtration through the glomerular membrane. Hydrogen ions undergo tubular secretion into the glomerular filtrate, whereas substances such as glucose, amino acids, and potassium ions are actively reabsorbed by the tubular membrane. Sublimation is a physical change from the solid directly to the gaseous state, and does not apply to the kidney or any other organ.

243. **The correct answer is (C).**

Stimulation of the sympathetic nervous system increases the heart rate, sweating, and blood pressure and dilates the pupils of the eyes. Stimulation of the parasympathetic nervous system produces opposite effects, that is, decreases the heart rate, sweating and blood pressure, as well as constriction of the pupils.

244. **The correct answer is (B).**

During heavy exercise, glycogen in the muscle breaks down to lactic acid faster than lactic acid can be oxidized, resulting in lactic acid accumulation.

245. **The correct answer is (C).**

Meiosis occurs during the formation of eggs or sperm, where a pair of cell divisions result in gametes with only half the number of chromosomes (haploid) as the other cells of the body. When two gametes unite in fertilization, the fusion of their nuclei reconstitutes the diploid number of chromosomes.

246. **The correct answer is (B).**

The physical appearance of any individual with respect to a given inherited trait is known as their phenotype. In contrast, an individual's genetic constitution, usually expressed in symbols, is called their genotype. Both recessive and heterozygous traits are related more to genotype rather than phenotype.

247. **The correct answer is (A).**

Sickle cell anemia is a condition where homozygous recessive genes are necessary for full development of the disease. If an individual has heterozygous recessive genes for the disease, that individual only shows sickle cell trait, but not the fully developed disease. Both beriberi and pellagra are diseases associated with vitamin deficiencies. Hypertension is usually of unknown etiology.

248. **The correct answer is (C).**

Intense exercise and training of an athlete can result in a decreased respiratory rate and an increase in the size in muscle fibers. However, there will be no increase in the number of muscle fibers, since this does not change after birth.

249. **The correct answer is (D).**

Spermatogonia (diploid) grow into primary spermatocytes (diploid) and then secondary spermatocytes (diploid) after the first meiotic division. Secondary spermatocytes become spermatids (haploid) after the second meiotic division.

250. **The correct answer is (A).**

An individual with type A-negative blood can receive blood from A-negative or O-negative donors. Rh positive blood cannot be given, since a transfusion reaction would result. B- and AB-type bloods cannot be given for the same reason.

251. The correct answer is (D).

The appendix, wisdom teeth, and coccygeal vertebrae (tail bone) serve no useful purpose in man; however, the pupils of the eyes are necessary for sight.

252. The correct answer is (C).

Graph C depicts a saturated reaction, as indicated by the initially straight lines for the product and substrate. The reaction proceeds to no substrate and all product, suggesting an irreversible reaction. Graph B indicates an unsaturated (curved lines) but irreversible (no substrate, all product after considerable time) reaction. Graph D represents an unsaturated reversible reaction, as shown by the initially curved line. This reaction also appears to be reversible, since the product and substrate appear to have reached an equilibrium. Thus, not all the substrate can be converted to product without some of the product reconverting to substrate.

253. The correct answer is (C).

The transport of oxygen and carbon dioxide in the blood depends largely on the amount of hemoglobin present in the red blood cell. Whole blood carries approximately 20 ml of oxygen and 60 ml of carbon dioxide per 100 ml. Plasma water carries only about 0.2–0.3 ml. of oxygen and carbon dioxide in each 100 ml. Plasma proteins carry essentially no oxygen.

254. The correct answer is (A).

Breeding between closely related individuals, commonly referred to as inbreeding, increases the proportion of homozygous individuals in a population, promoting the occurrence or double recessive traits of congenital anomalies. Some genetic disorders including muscular dystrophy and red-green color blindness are known to be sex-linked defective traits.

255. The correct answer is (A).

Beneficial associations or interactions between two species of animals include commensalism, protocooperation, and mutualism. Negative interactions between two species include amensalism, parasitism, and predation.

256. The correct answer is (D).

This question is similar to Question 252. Graph D shows unsaturated reaction characteristics (initially curved lines).

257. The correct answer is (B).

Albumin (~5 g/100 ml of plasma) is the plasma protein most responsible for the osmotic pressure. Both fibrinogen and gammaglobulin are plasma proteins that contribute to the colloid osmotic pressure, but to a considerably lesser degree. Hemoglobin is a red pigment responsible for the transport of oxygen and carbon dioxide in the blood.

258. The correct answer is (C).

Only red blood cells carry hemoglobin, the substance responsible for oxygen and carbon dioxide transport.

259. **The correct answer is (D).**

Plasma cells, derived from lymphocytes, produce and secrete antibodies. Thrombocytes, important in initiating the clotting of blood, are formed by the fragmentation of giant cells, megakaryocytes, in the red bone marrow. Neutrophils are important in taking up bacteria and dead tissue cells by phagocytosis.

260. **The correct answer is (A).**

Cyanide is routinely employed as an inhibitor of enzymatic reactions. Therefore, treatment with cyanide will arrest the enzymatic reaction, and substrate will not be changed to product (Graph A).

261. **The correct answer is (C).**

The hemoglobin in the red blood cell has a high capacity for binding both oxygen and carbon dioxide. A lack of hemoglobin (anemia) results in a decreased capacity for oxygen and carbon dioxide transport.

262. **The correct answer is (A).**

Albumin (5 g/100 ml of plasma) is approximately 2.5 times more abundant than globulin (2 g/100 ml of plasma). Fibrinogen and immunoglobulins are present in small amounts compared to albumin.

263. **The correct answer is (D).**

Whereas decreased oxygen delivery to tissues (or a low blood oxygen concentration) will increase the number of red blood cells, increased carbon dioxide concentration will not. Changes in the number of red blood cells appear to be associated with changes in blood oxygen tension rather than in blood carbon dioxide tension.

264. **The correct answer is (B).**

Sweating, increased metabolism, and vasodilation of the blood vessels help transfer body heat to the surrounding environment. Increased muscle tone does not significantly increase heat loss.

265. **The correct answer is (C).**

Urea and creatinine normally pass through the kidney in the glomerular filtrate. Conversely, normally all the glucose in the glomerular filtrate is actively reabsorbed by the kidney in the normal individual. Glucose can be found in the urine when the blood glucose concentration is abnormally elevated (> 180 mg %), as in uncontrolled diabetes.

266. **The correct answer is (D).**

The reticular activating system is involved in the control of sleep, wakefulness, attentiveness, and behavior, but does not actively participate in regulating the volume of body fluids. The baroreceptors and vasomotor center of the brain work together to increase the flow of blood to the glomeruli of the kidneys, resulting in increased glomerular filtration and formation of urine. The osmoreceptors control the amount of water reabsorbed from the tubular filtrate of the kidneys by the secretion of antidiuretic hormone.

267. **The correct answer is (C).**

The axon and dendrites are components of the neuron. The dendrites constitute that part of the neuron specialized for receiving excitation, whereas the axon is the part specialized to distribute or conduct excitation away from the dendritic zone. Nerves are usually composed of collections of axons.

268. **The correct answer is (A).**

The rate of conduction increases as the diameter of the axon increases, because there is less resistance to the action potential. Thus, larger nerve fibers have a faster rate of conduction than smaller ones. Myelin sheaths usually increase the rate of conduction by insulating the action potential on the axon from the external environment, again decreasing resistance.

269. **The correct answer is (B).**

The autonomic nervous system, composed of both sympathetic and parasympathetic nerves, is responsible for the involuntary activities of the body. Motor impulses reach the effector organ from the brain or spinal cord through a series of motor neurons comprising the corticospinal (pyramidal) and extracorticospinal (extrapyramidal).

270. **The correct answer is (D).**

Thyroxine is an iodinated derivative of the amino acid tyrosine. Other hormones derived from amino acids include melatonin and epinephrine. Prostaglandins are derivatives of 20-carbon unsaturated fatty acids, whereas estradiol and testosterone are derived from cholesterol.

271. **The correct answer is (C).**

A single muscle twitch is caused by an initiating action potential; however, there is a latent period after the generation of the action potential and initiation of the muscle twitch. After the latent period, the muscle contracts and then relaxes, followed by a refractory period in which the muscle will not respond to another action potential.

272. **The correct answer is (D).**

The nervous system provides instantaneous control of a body function, whereas hormones usually take a relatively long time (hours or days) to regulate a body function.

273. **The correct answer is (A).**

Progesterone is secreted by the corpus luteum and acts with estradiol to regulate the estrous and menstrual cycles. Vasopressin, secreted by the hypothalamus, stimulates the contraction of smooth muscles and has an antidiuretic action on kidney tubules. Aldosterone regulates metabolism of sodium and potassium and is secreted by the adrenal cortex.

274. **The correct answer is (C).**

The rods of the retina are responsible for peripheral, achromatic, and poor detail vision. Central, color, and detail vision is a function of the cones of the retina.

275. **The correct answer is (A).**

The rate of lymph flow is much slower (~100 ml/hr) than blood flow (~5 liter/min) in man and most animal species.

Explanatory Answers
Test 4: Chemistry

276. **The correct answer is (D).**

Alkanes are saturated hydrocarbons containing only carbon and hydrogen. They are usually straight-chained compounds and the carbon atom utilizes four sp^3 hybrid orbitals, forming a tetrahedral arrangement. Each bond angle is 109.5°, and the general formula is C_nH_{2n+2}; for example, when there is one C atom, then there are four H atoms, as in methane. Alkenes have the general formula C_nH_{2n}.

277. **The correct answer is (B).**

With regard to phenol, electron-releasing substituents (e.g., —CH_3) will decrease its acidity and lower the K_a. An electron-attracting substituent (e.g., —NO_2) will withdraw the ring electrons, relatively, and increase the acidity of phenol, resulting in a higher K_a. Thus, a nitro substituent in the ortho position will increase the K_a, whereas a methyl substituent in the same position would lower the K_a. Furthermore, the —OH substituent is strongly ortho and para directing.

278. **The correct answer is (B).**

Using the pH concept, we have $pH = -\log[H^+] = \log\left[\dfrac{1}{[H^+]}\right]$.

Furthermore, $pOH = \log\left[\dfrac{1}{[OH^-]}\right]$, and $[H^+][OH^-]$ equals 10^{-14}.

From these relations, $pH + pOH = 14$.

279. **The correct answer is (A).**

Hematite (Fe_2O_3) has a molecular weight of 160. The percentage of elemental iron in hematite is given as follows:

$$\frac{2Fe}{Fe_2O_3} = \frac{2(56)}{160} \times 100\%$$
$$= 70\%$$

Note that there are two atoms of iron in Fe_2O_3.

280. **The correct answer is (B).**

$$3H_2 \quad + \quad N_2 \quad \rightarrow \quad 2NH_3$$
$$\text{(3 liters)} \quad \text{(1 liter)} \quad \text{(2 liters)}$$

Setting up a direct proportion, that is,

$$\frac{2 \text{ liters of } NH_3}{2 \text{ liters of } H_2} = \frac{20 \text{ liters of } NH_3}{x \text{ liters of } H_2}$$

and solving for x will give an answer of 30 liters.

281. The correct answer is (B).

The volume occupied by the gram-molecular weight of a gas under standard temperature and pressure conditions (i.e., 0°C and 760 mmHg) is called the gram-molecular volume. Hence, 1 mole of any gas under these conditions will occupy a volume of 22.4 liters. Be aware that 1 mole of the same gas may occupy a different volume at some other combination of temperature and pressure.

282. The correct answer is (B).

The molecular weight of CO_2 is 44 g (i.e., 12 + 32). Thus, the gram-molecular weight of CO_2 is 44 g, which occupies 22.4 liters at standard temperature and pressure. Therefore, the weight of 1 liter of CO_2

equals $\dfrac{(44\ g)}{(22.4\ liters)} = 1.9$ g. Since there are 2 liters of CO_2, the weight is 4 g.

283. The correct answer is (A).

In acetylene, carbon forms two *sp* hybrid orbitals and thus enables itself to bind to two hydrogen atoms in a sigma bond. The carbon-carbon triple bond, however, is made up of one sigma bond and two pi bonds.

284. The correct answer is (C).

The carbon in methane (CH_4) and the oxygen in water (H_2O) both form sp^3 hybrid orbitals. For carbon, the sp^3 hybridization results in four hybrid orbitals in which the axes are directed toward the corners of a tetrahedron. In the formation of water, oxygen bonds with two hydrogen atoms via its two unpaired electrons. The water molecule still has a tetrahedral shape; two corners are occupied by hydrogen atoms and the rest is occupied by the unshared pairs of electrons.

285. The correct answer is (B).

In chemistry, the structural formula (e.g., $C_6H_{12}O_6$) reveals the numbers and types of atoms present in a molecule. In general, if not always, the arrangement of the different atoms can also be deduced from an examination of the structural formula. However, the structural formula of a molecule bears no relationship to the gram-molecular volume occupied by the gram-molecular weight of a gas under standard conditions.

286. The correct answer is (B).

A knowledge of the chemical and physical properties of organic and inorganic compounds is important in understanding their chemical behavior. Organic compounds do exist as isomers and decompose upon heating at lower temperatures. They are also soluble in other organic solvents; that is, like dissolves like. However, organic compounds do not react with each other faster than inorganic compounds would.

287. The correct answer is (C).

In radioactive disintegration, the emission of a beta particle does not change the atomic weight of the nucleus emitting the beta particle. This is due to the fact that the weight of a beta particle is extremely small. However, the atomic number increases by 1 and is thought to be the result of the breakdown of a neutron to a proton and an electron (beta particle). An alpha particle is a helium nucleus, and its emission, in contrast to that of a beta particle, results in a decrease of 4 units of atomic weight and 2 units of atomic number.

288. The correct answer is (C).

The artificial conversion of one element into another (e.g., nitrogen into oxygen) is termed transmutation. Radioactive decay can occur spontaneously, resulting in the disintegration of the parent nucleus, with the consequent production of one or more daughter nuclei. This process is usually accompanied by the emanation (i.e., emission) of gamma rays. *Transformation* is a nonspecific term for changes in physical form.

289. The correct answer is (C).

Gamma rays are high-energy X-rays of very short wavelength that travel with the speed of light. Compared to alpha and beta rays, gamma rays are the most penetrating of the radiations emitted by radioactive compounds. Since they have no electrical charge, magnetic or electrical fields do not affect their path.

290. The correct answer is (D).

Atomic fusion is the process of combining atoms to form elements of higher atomic weight. Frequently tremendous energy is released during this process. Atomic fission is the process of splitting an atomic nucleus, which also results in the release of large amounts of energy. The process of electron capture results from the conversion of an orbital electron to a neutron, and the energy therein is negligible compared to that of atomic fusion and fission.

291. The correct answer is (D).

Alcohols have the general formula ROH. While methanol and ethanol are the simplest and most easily recognized alcohols, glycerine is also an alcohol, even though it has three hydroxyl groups. Glycerine (or glycerol) is thus a polyalcohol and is widely used in pharmaceutical manufacturing. Sodium hydroxide (NaOH) is a base and not an alcohol. Remember that alcohols are organic compounds in which the hydroxyl group has been substituted for one or more hydrogen atoms in a hydrocarbon.

292. The correct answer is (A).

Hydrogen chloride gas has a pungent smell, is extremely soluble in water, and reacts with ammonia to form white fumes of ammonium chloride. It is a colorless gas, but is not lighter than air. The density of the gas is greater than 1 g/cm^3 and is about 25% heavier than air.

293. The correct answer is (D).

The halogen elements are fluorine, chlorine, bromine, iodine, and astatine. They comprise group VIIA of the periodic table. Note that these elements end in the suffix *-ine*; however, this does not mean that turpentine or nicotine belong to the halogen family.

294. The correct answer is (A).

It can be stated that 1 Eq of any chemical is that quantity that is equivalent to 1 mole of replaceable hydrogen ions in an acid-base reaction. Thus, 1 mole of HCl contains 1 mole of replaceable hydrogen, and thus HCl has 1 Eq/mole. $HC_2H_3O_2$ is the formula for acetic acid, CH_3COOH. Clearly, only one hydrogen ionizes, and therefore acetic acid has 1 Eq/mole.

295. The correct answer is (D).

Avogadro's law determines the relation between the properties of gases. In essence, it states that equal volumes of different gases at the same temperature and pressure contain the same number of molecules. Hence, if one keeps the temperature and pressure constant, the volume of any gas is proportional to its mass, and therefore to the number of gas molecules. Note that Charles' law states that the volume of a gas is directly proportional to the absolute temperature, provided that pressure remains constant. Boyle's law relates the pressure and volume of a gas at constant temperature.

296. The correct answer is (C).

There is one chiral center and thus 2 possible isomers or 2 configurations.

297. The correct answer is (B).

R from the Latin rectus, meaning right and S from the Latin sinister, meaning left.

298. The correct answer is (D).

If one assumes complete ionization, 58.5 mg of sodium chloride will supply 23 mg of sodium ions. Similarly, to give 100 mg of sodium ions, it is required to supply $\dfrac{(100 \times 58.5)}{23} = 254$ mg of sodium chloride crystals.

299. The correct answer is (D).

One mEq of sodium chloride is equal to its gram-equivalent weight divided by 1000. Hence, 1 mEq of sodium chloride equals 58.5 mg of sodium chloride and 2 mEq equals 117 mg. The concentration of this solution is 117 mg/ml.

300. The correct answer is (A).

The milliequivalent is used primarily by the health profession to express the concentration of electrolytes in solution. Since Mr. Smith weighs 60 kg, he should receive 2 × 60 mEq of sodium chloride. One mEq of sodium chloride equals 58.5 mg of salt. Therefore, Mr. Smith requires 2 × 60 × 58.5 mg of sodium chloride. The answer is 7020 mg, or 7 g.

301. The correct answer is (A).

Percent (%) means parts per hundred on a weight basis. Hence, a 0.9% solution translates to 0.9 g of sodium chloride per 100 ml of solution. Mr. Smith requires 7 g, which is $\dfrac{(7 \times 100 \text{ ml})}{0.9}$ of solution. This comes out to 777 ml of a 0.9% solution of sodium chloride.

302. The correct answer is (A).

The pharmacist must be well versed with the different units used to express the strength or concentration of a particular drug in solution. This problem relates to a solution of sodium chloride that is half the strength ordered. Hence, twice the volume must be supplied to give the same amount of sodium chloride ordered, that is, 777 ml × 2 = 1.5 liters.

303. **The correct answer is (B).**

Osmotic pressure is directly affected by the total number of particles in solution. If one assumes complete dissociation, 1 mole of sodium chloride is composed of 2 mOsm of total particles (i.e., Na^+ and Cl^-).

304. **The correct answer is (D).**

Osmotic activity is a function of the total number of particles present in a given solution, be they electrolytes or nonelectrolytes. Electrolytes, generally, will dissociate into their component ions, and hence the number of particles in solution will increase.

305. **The correct answer is (C).**

This question illustrates the need to convert different units to arrive at the answer. One millimole of sodium chloride is equal to 2 mOsm of the salt. One millimole of sodium chloride is 58.5 mg . Since a 0.9% solution has 0.9 g (or 900 mg) of sodium chloride per 100 ml of solution, 900 mg of this sodium chloride is equal to $\dfrac{900}{58.5}$ or 15.4 mmole of sodium chloride. Now, since 1 mmole of sodium chloride is equal to 2 mOsm, 15.4 mmole equals 15.4×2 mOsm of sodium chloride. The answer is 31 mOsm.

306. **The correct answer is (C).**

Hydrogen has an atomic number and an atomic weight of 1. Hence, it has one proton and one electron, which reside in the nucleus and K shell, respectively. Hydrogen does not have a neutron. The hydrogen isotopes deuterium and tritium have one and two neutrons in the nucleus, respectively.

307. **The correct answer is (D).**

This problem relates to the concept of atomic weight and atomic number. The total number of protons equals the number of electrons in the shells. Beryllium has four electrons, and therefore four protons. The total number of protons equals the atomic number, and therefore beryllium has an atomic number of 4. The total number of protons and neutrons comprises the atomic weight of the element. Beryllium has an atomic weight of 9, since it has five neutrons and four protons.

308. **The correct answer is (B).**

Mercury forms bivalent mercuric (Hg^{2+}) and bivalent mercurous (Hg_2^{2+}) compounds, even though mercury has a valence of 2 and 1, respectively. Mercurous oxide is Hg_2O. Hg_2O_3, Hg_3O_2, and HgO_2 compounds are unknown.

309. **The correct answer is (A).**

HNO_2 is nitrous acid. Nitronous acid, nitrate acid, and nitrite acid do not exist.

310. **The correct answer is (C).**

The reverse of synthesis is decomposition, that is, the breakdown of a compound AB to yield an element A and an element B.

311. The correct answer is (C).

When a particle is oxidized, it loses electrons. Therefore, oxidation is associated with electron loss. Conversely, reduction is associated with electron gain. Since oxidation and reduction processes occur simultaneously, loss and/or gain of electrons is to be expected. An oxidized particle therefore loses its (valence) electrons, which results in an increase in valence number.

312. The correct answer is (C).

This is an exercise in the law of conservation of matter. Examination of the equation will show that the number of molecules of the reactants must equal the number of molecules of the products, that is,

$$2ABC_3 \quad \rightarrow \quad 2AB + 3C_2$$

Reactant	=	Product
2A		2A
2B		2B
6C		6C

313. The correct answer is (D).

The oxygen molecule is diatomic (O_2). Ozone is a triatomic molecule (O_3) of oxygen; its properties are different from those of oxygen.

314. The correct answer is (A).

It is common knowledge that oxygen gas is combustible; however, it cannot be overemphasized that oxygen *supports* combustion and does not burn by itself. Its lack of odor and color does not help in its quick identification.

315. The correct answer is (D).

Hydrogen peroxide is H_2O_2. The word *peroxide* means that it contains one more oxygen atom than would normally be expected. Water (H_2O) is the simplest molecule formed between the atoms of oxygen and hydrogen. Two molecules of hydrogen peroxide decompose via the following reaction, yielding two molecules of water and one molecule of oxygen: $2H_2O_2 \rightarrow 2H_2O + O_2$

316. The correct answer is (C).

This problem deals with the concept of density. Since the gram is defined as the mass of 1 cm³ (approximately 1 ml) of water at 4°C, water has a density of 1 g/ml; 5000 ml of water weigh 5000 g.

317. The correct answer is (D).

The student is expected to be familiar with the different units used in expressing the quantity of a given solute in a quantity of solvent or total solution. Molarity (*M*) is defined as the number of moles of solute per liter of solution. In contrast, molality is the number of moles of solute in 1 kg of solvent. You should also be aware that normality (*N*) is defined as the number of equivalents of solute per liter of solution.

318.   The correct answer is (B).

The molecular weight of NaOH is 40. Hence, 40 g of NaOH are equivalent to 1 mole of NaOH. Molarity is defined as the number of moles of solute per liter of solution. Therefore, 1 mole of NaOH dissolved in 1 liter of solution is a 1 M solution. Dissolving 1 mole in 400 ml would give a higher molarity, that is, an increase by a factor of 2.5.

319.   The correct answer is (C).

If you are still unclear about moles and molarity by the time you get to this question, a review is required. One mole of sodium hydroxide equals 40 g dissolved in 1 liter of solution. A 5 M (molar) solution would mean 5 × 40 g of sodium hydroxide dissolved in 1 liter of solution. Hence, 125 ml of this solution would contain (125 × 5 × 40) /1000 of sodium hydroxide. The number of moles would now be easy to calculate: Just divide (125 × 5 × 40) g /1000 by 40 g/mole. The answer is 0.625 mole.

320.   The correct answer is (C).

Since 125 ml of a 5 M solution contains 0.625 mole of sodium hydroxide, then 0.625 mole × 40 g/ mole of sodium hydroxide yields 25 g of this base.

321.   The correct answer is (A).

A liter of pure water weighs 1 kg, if one assumes that water has a density of 1 g/ml. The molecular weight of water is 18 g/mole. One liter of pure water, therefore, contains $\dfrac{(1000\ g)}{18\ g\,/\,mole}$ or 55.5 moles; 55.5 moles 18 g/mole of water in a solution represents a molarity of 55.5.

322.   The correct answer is (D).

Colligative properties of solutions depend on the amount and concentration of the solute(s) in the solution. Hence boiling point, vapor pressure, and freezing point are all colligative properties. Specific gravity, which compares the weights of substances to that of water, is not a colligative property.

323.   The correct answer is (A).

Acid and base strengths are frequently expressed by pH values. The pH value of any number is defined as the negative logarithm (base 10) of that number; that is, if $x = 10^n$, then $\log x = n$ and the pH of x is $-n$. Since pH = $-\log[H^+]$ = $-\log[1]$, pH = 0. Note that a pH of 0 is not neutral. A pH of 7 represents neutrality.

324.   The correct answer is (D).

Since pOH + pH = 14 and pH = O, pOH equals 14. This would represent a very basic (strongly alkaline) solution.

325.   The correct answer is (A).

As indicated before, the pH value gives some idea of the strength of an acid or base. The higher the pH value, the lower the hydrogen ion concentration. A higher pH means that the substance is less acidic and more basic.

326. The correct answer is (A).

Methane (CH_4) is the simplest saturated hydrocarbon of the alkane series. It is explosive when mixed with air, is the active component of natural gas, and is otherwise called marsh gas. Owing to its saturated character, methane is not important in addition reactions, but it will undergo substitution reactions.

327. The correct answer is (C).

Esters have the general formula RCOOR. Ethyl acetate is $C_2H_5COOCH_3$. Nitroglycerine and methyl salicylate are both esters. Sodium formate (NaCOOH) is the salt of an organic acid and is therefore not an ester.

328. The correct answer is (B).

Glucose is a monosaccharide. Dextran and cellulose are polysaccharides. Glyceryl stearate is a fatty acid and is widely employed in making soaps, for example, sodium stearate.

329. The correct answer is (A).

Rayon, nylon, and Orlon are all synthetic fibers. Nylon is a synthetic protein, Orlon is a polyester fiber, and rayon is regenerated cellulose; however, cellulose is a nonsynthetic fiber.

330. The correct answer is (A).

Werner Heisenberg showed that when one attempts to simultaneously debermine the position and momentum of an electron, an unavoidable uncertainty in both these parameters is created that cannot be resolved. Louis de Broglie advanced the hypothesis that electrons have wavelike characteristics, Planck is responsible for the foundations of quantum theory, and Bohr is known for his electronic theory of the atom.

331. The correct answer is (A).

Four quantum numbers are necessary in order to fully characterize the electronic wave functions; these are n (the principle quantum number), l (the azimuthal quantum number), m (the magnetic quantum number), and s (the spin quantum number).

332. The correct answer is (B).

Pauli's exclusion principle clearly demonstrates that an atom cannot exist in a state where two electrons in the same orbital have the same four quantum numbers. This principle is important when more and more electrons are added to the orbitals of the atoms in the periodic table.

333. The correct answer is (B).

The student is expected to remember the atomic numbers of the first 10 elements in the periodic table. Oxygen has eight electrons and its orbitals are filled according to a $1s^2 2s^2 2p^4$ electronic configuration. You should remember the minimum (or maximum) number of electrons that can occupy any orbital. These $s, p, d,$ and f orbitals can be completely filled by 2, 6, 10 and 14 electrons, respectively.

334. The correct answer is (B).

Carbon has six protons and, therefore, six electrons; however, its atomic weight is 12; that is, it has six protons and six neutrons. Hence, carbon has six protons, six electrons, and six neutrons. Remember that the atomic number is equal to the number of protons (or electrons) and that the atomic weight is the number of protons *and* neutrons in the nucleus.

335. **The correct answer is (B).**

The $1s^2 2s^2 2p^2$ electronic distribution translates to six orbital electrons. Hence, this element has six electrons and therefore six protons. Carbon has six protons and six electrons. Beryllium has four electrons, helium has two, and oxygen has eight. The element in question is carbon.

336. **The correct answer is (D).**

Isotopes are atoms of elements having the same number of electrons, the same chemical characteristics, and the same valence. However, isotopes differ in their mass, that is, in the number of neutrons in the nucleus, for example hydrogen (no neutrons) and tritium (two neutrons).

337. **The correct answer is (A).**

Carbon-12 (ordinary carbon) has six electrons, six protons, and six neutrons. Carbon-14 is an isotope of carbon and differs only in mass (i.e., neutron number). Hence, carbon-14 has two extra neutrons when compared to natural carbon. In summary, carbon-12 has six electrons, six protons, and six neutrons; carbon-14 has six electrons, six protons, and six neutrons.

338. **The correct answer is (B).**

Gamma-ray decay is associated primarily with the emission of electromagnetic radiation, that is, photons. The internal rearrangement of the atom is responsible for gamma-ray emission, and there are no changes in the nuclear mass (i.e., the number of protons and neutrons) of the atom. Alpha decay is associated with a decrease of 4 units of atomic weight.

339. **The correct answer is (C).**

The angstrom (A°) is 1×10^{-10} m, or 1×10^{-8} cm, the average radius of an atom.

340. **The correct answer is (D).**

The prefix *pyro-* indicates loss of water. In this example, a molecule of water is lost from two molecules of orthophosphoric acid to form pyrophosphoric acid. The prefixes *hypo-* and *per-* refer, respectively, to the lowest and highest oxidation states. The prefix for the highest hydrated form is *ortho-*.

341. **The correct answer is (A).**

Lead exists in the divalent (+2) and tetravalent (+4) oxidation states, where it is called the plumbus and plumbic ion, respectively. Copper also exists in two oxidation states, monovalent (+I) and divalent (+2).

342. **The correct answer is (B).**

The alkaline-earth metals comprise group IIA of the periodic table. Phosphorus is not one of the elements in this group. Gypsum and plaster of paris are sulfate salts of calcium, the most abundant and useful element of group IIA. Plaster of paris is used to make plaster and surgical casts.

343. **The correct answer is (C).**

Hydrogen sulfide gas not only smells obnoxious to the user, but it is also extremely toxic. It is a colorless gas, denser than air, and somewhat soluble in water; hence, the preparation and use of this gas should be carefully monitored.

344. The correct answer is (D).

CH_3COOH follows the general formula RCOOH, which represents an organic acid. This particular organic acid is acetic acid, commonly called vinegar. Aqua fortis is the common name for nitric acid. Aqua regia is a mixture of nitric and hydrochloric acids, while muriatic acid is commercially produced hydrochloric acid.

345. The correct answer is (D).

Baking soda is sodium bicarbonate, $NaHCO_3$. Sodium carbonate (Na_2CO_3) is washing soda and is used as a water softener. $Na_2B_4O_7$ is borax, while magnesium sulfate ($MgSO_4$) is known as Epsom salts.

346. The correct answer is (C).

HOCl is hypochlorous acid, formed from the initial reaction of chlorine gas and water. Most bleaching agents (e.g., Clorox) act by the release of hypochlorous acid into solution. Chloroform is an organic solvent ($CHCl_3$). Brine is the form of sodium chloride found in combination with sea water, while tincture of iodine is an alcoholic preparation contining iodine.

347. The correct answer is (B).

Alkenes have double bonds. This double bond is made up of one pi bond and one sigma bond. In organic chemistry there are no alpha bonds, but there are alpha-designated carbon atoms.

348. The correct answer is (A).

$RCONH_2$ are amides, the simplest member being formamide ($HCONH_2$). Acid anhydrides have the general formula $(RCO)_2O$, amines are generally RNH_2, while azides have the general formula $RCON_3$.

349. The correct answer is (C).

An enzyme usually has the suffix *-ase*, sugar usually ends in *-ose*, while a carboxyl group would end in *-ate*.

350. The correct answer is (A).

A tertiary (3°) alcohol has all of its alcohol carbon hydrogens substituted for other organic substituents; a secondary (2°) alcohol has only one hydrogen attached to the alcohol carbon; and a primary (1°) alcohol has only two hydrogens attached to the alcohol carbon. CH_3OH is methanol, which has only hydrogen attached to the alcohol carbon.

351. The correct answer is (B).

Vinyl usually refers to the $CH_2 = CH$ radical. Thus methyl vinyl ketone is $CH_3COCH = CH_2$. Ethyl vinyl ketone is $CH_3CH_2COCH = CH_2$. Butyric acid is $CH_3CH_2CH_2COOH$, whereas $CH_3OCH_2CH = CH_2$ is methyl allyl ether.

352. The correct answer is (D).

An organic acid is usually identified by the longest hydrocarbon chain, with the carboxyl carbon as carbon number 1. Changing the suffix from *-ane* to *-ol* would make it an alcohol and not an acid.

353. **The correct answer is (D).**

$CH_3(CH_2)_8CH_3$ has 10 carbon atoms; hence, it is called decane. Nonane has nine carbon atoms, while octane has only eight. Undecane is $C_{11}H_{24}$, and there are thus 11 carbon atoms in this saturated hydrocarbon.

354. **The correct answer is (C).**

Atoms in double- or triple-bonded systems are rigid and not free to rotate around these bonds. Furthermore, ring systems have an aromatic character, and the atoms in these systems are also not free to rotate around their bonds. Only atoms connected by single bonds rotate around their sigma bonds.

355. **The correct answer is (B).**

The carbonium ions, by definition, are atoms that contain a carbon atom with only six electrons. They are classified as primary, secondary, and tertiary ions, as in the classification of the organic alcohols. Since the stability of a carbonium ion is greatly increased by charge dispersal, a tertiary carbonium ion, which has three alkyl groups, is more stable than a secondary carbonium ion, which has two alkyl groups. The more stable the carbonium ion, the more easily it is formed.

356. **The correct answer is (D).**

Benzene is a planar molecule; that is, all its atoms lie in the same plane. There are pi electron clouds above and below the plane of the ring, making it a rigid molecule with the formula C_6H_6. Each carbon atom lies at an angle of a regular six-sided figure, or hexagon. The bond angle is therefore 120°.

357. **The correct answer is (C).**

Aldehyde and ketones have the carbonyl ($—C = 0$) functional group. The carbonyl carbon is joined to three other atoms by sigma bonds; there is also an overlap of a pi bond. The carbon hybridization orbitals are sp^2, and the molecule is planar, with bond angles of 120°.

358. **The correct answer is (B).**

With regard to chemical reactivity and nucleophilic displacement, nucleophilic substitution occurs more readily at an acyl carbon (i.e., —RCO) than at a saturated carbon. Hence, a compound having a carbonyl group would be more prone to undergo nucleophilic substitution, for example, amides would be more prone than amines, acid chlorides more than alkyl chlorides, and esters more than ethers.

359. **The correct answer is (A).**

Glycols are polyalcohols, usually containing two hydroxyl groups. These are saturated compounds, the simplest being ethylene glycol, CH_2OHCH_2OH. The suffix *-ol* should remind you that we are dealing with alcohols.

360. **The correct answer is (B).**

The Grignard reagent is unique owing to its high reactivity. Its general formula is RMgX, and it is formed by reacting an alkyl halide with metallic magnesium in ether. The carbon-magnesium bond is highly polar but distinctly covalent (i.e., sharing of electrons); however, the magnesium-halogen bond is ionic in character.

361. The correct answer is (C).

Organic molecules are such that reactants must be optically active in order for the products to be optically active. The converse, that is, the relation between inactive reactants and inactive products, is also correct. However, the products of optically active reactants may not show such activity, and this is due to racemic modification of the isomers.

362. The correct answer is (D).

CH_4 is methane, and $—CH_3$ is the methyl radical of this alkane. CH_2 or methylene exists as a discrete molecule and is highly reactive. Methanol is formaldehyde, the former being the International Union of Pure and Applied Chemistry (IUPAC) nomenclature and the latter being the common name. Mesyl is the shortened form of the methyl sulfonyl radical and deals with sulfonic acid chemistry.

363. The correct answer is (D).

The Diels-Alder reaction is important because the end product of the reactants, a diene and a dienophile, is a six-membered ring. The diene usually possesses electron-releasing groups, while the dienophile (an $\alpha\beta$-unsaturated carbonyl compound) is associated with electron-withdrawing functional groups. Note that the Diels-Alder reaction is a reaction between a conjugated diene and an α-unsaturated carbonyl compound.

364. The correct answer is (A).

Disaccharides, on hydrolysis, yield two monosaccharides. Sucrose (cane sugar) will yield glucose and fructose. Maltose (malt sugar) will yield two molecules of glucose, while lactose (milk sugar) will yield glucose and galactose. Amylose is a water-soluble fraction of starch, a polysaccharide.

365. The correct answer is (C).

Amino acids have the general formula $RCHNH_2COOH$. The amino acid with the simplest structure is NH_2CH_2COOH, or glycine. Tyrosine is an aromatic amino acid, whereas arginine is a basic amino acid. Methionine is an amino acid containing an atom of sulfur.

366. The correct answer is (B).

Aryl halides are compounds in which the halogens are attached directly to the aromatic ring, for example, bromobenzene (C_6H_5Br). Alkyl halides are not only the saturated form of the halogen-containing compounds, for they also compose the substituted alkyl group, for example, vinyl chloride.

367. The correct answer is (D).

The catalytic addition of oxygen to ethylene ($CH_2 = CH_2$) results in the formation of ethylene oxide, which has the structure

$$CH_2 \overset{}{\underset{O}{\diagdown\diagup}} CH_2$$

Ethylene oxide is therefore an epoxide, whereas ethylene is an alkene.

368. **The correct answer is (C).**

Amines have the general formula RNH_2. Primary amines have the formula RNH_2, secondary amines have the formula R_2NH, and tertiary amines have the formula R_3N. RNH is an amine radical and lacks either an R group or a hydrogen atom.

369. **The correct answer is (C).**

One hundred percent alcohol (or 200 proof alcohol) is absolute alcohol or water-free alcohol. Methanol is synonymous with wood alcohol. Absolute alcohol absorbs various amounts of water from the atmosphere and must be stored accordingly.

370. **The correct answer is (A).**

The simplest member of the fused-ring hydrocarbon family is naphthalene, which has two benzene rings. Anthracene has three fused benzene rings, just like phenanthrene.

371. **The correct answer is (B).**

CH_3OH is the formula for an organic alcohol commonly known as methanol. Menthone is a long-chained organic compound (i.e., a terpene) with a keto group, whereas mesitol is trimethyl phenol, an alkyl-substituted aryl alcohol. Menthol is a cyclic alcohol derived from mint oils.

372. **The correct answer is (C).**

Tollen's reagent contains $Ag(NH_3)_2^+$, the silver ammonium ion. Oxidation of an aldehyde to an acid is accompanied by the formation of a silver mirror. The latter is the result of the reduction of the soluble silver ion to yield free silver metal.

373. **The correct answer is (D).**

Ammonia has the formula NH_3. Nitrogen uses four sp^3 orbitals in forming this molecule; they are directed toward the corners of a regular tetrahedron, with one orbital containing a pair of electrons. The other three each contain a single electron.

374. **The correct answer is (B).**

By converting an organic acid to an acid chloride, we can produce a substance from which we can form esters and amides. Acid chlorides are much more reactive than their original acid and are therefore quite useful. Because of their reactivity, thionyl chloride and the chlorides of phosphorus are commonly employed in the preparation of acid chlorides. Note that these compounds have sulfur or phosphorus as the inorganic element. Ethyl chloride is a substituted halogenated hydrocarbon and plays no role in the preparation of such acid chlorides.

375. **The correct answer is (A).**

All monosaccharides are reducing sugars, that is, they reduce Tollen's or Fehling's reagent. These monosaccharides can be aldo or keto sugars. Glucose is a monosaccharide and hence a reducing sugar. Most disaccharides are reducing sugars as well. Even though sucrose is a disaccharide, it does not, however, reduce Tollen's or Fehling's solution.

Explanatory Answers
Test 5: Reading Comprehension

376. **The correct answer is (D).**

The answer to this question is found in line **7** of the paragraph. An intramuscular solution is given intramuscularly rather than intravenously.

377. **The correct answer is (B).**

The answer is found in lines **19 and 20** of the paragraph. There are several variables, including the answer, that affect the rate of flow of medication: gravity, temperature, and possibly the equipment itself.

378. **The correct answer is (A).**

The answer is found in lines **22–25**: "When the rate of flow is critical, such as in pediatric patients or in parenteral nutrition, an infusion pump may be needed to ensure the proper flow of solution into the patient."

379. **The correct answer is (B).**

The answer is found in lines **1–4** of the paragraph: "Before the intravenous administration of a medication, it is essential to check the medication, the dose, fluid in which the drug is to be given, and time of administration against the patient's chart."

380. **The correct answer is (B).**

The answer is found in lines **1–3** of the paragraph. Bronchoconstrictors do not appear in the list of items in which adrenergic agents are commonly found.

381. **The correct answer is (C).**

The answer is found in lines **16–18** of the paragraph: "General anesthetics producing parasympathetic and sympathetic imbalance may cause pupillary block."

382. **The correct answer is (B).**

The answer is found in lines **9–12** of the paragraph: "It is important to note, however, that these agents will elevate the intraocular pressure by narrowing the anterior chamber angle when instilled into eyes of angle closure patients."

383. **The correct answer is (C).**

The answer is found in lines **9–11** of the paragraph: "Adrenergic agents such as epinephrine and phenylephrine have been used ocularly to treat open-angle glaucoma."

384. **The correct answer is (D).**

The answer is found in lines **18–20** of the paragraph. "To prevent this complication, topical pilocarpine at 1% may be instilled into the eye 1 hr prior to anesthesia."

385. **The correct answer is (C).**

The answer is found in lines **6 and 7** of the paragraph: "Ventricular tachycardia usually requires intravenous therapy."

386. **The correct answer is (C).**

The answer is found in lines **14–16** of the paragraph: "Doses of 50-100 mg of diphenylhydantoin, up to a maximum of 1.0 g, may be administered intravenously every 5 minutes."

387. **The correct answer is (A).**

The answer is found in lines **22 and 23** of the paragraph: "Generally, cardiovascular complications can be avoided with an infusion rate of 20-50 mg/min."

388. **The correct answer is (D).**

The answer is found in lines **18–21** of the paragraph: "Single intravenous doses of 300 mg or more produce a more marked hypotension (20-45 mmHg) and also lead to subtherapeutic diphenylhydantoin plasma levels."

389. **The correct answer is (B).**

The answer is found in lines **7–11** of the paragraph: "There appears to be no indication in this situation for intrammuscular injections, because the drug is slowly and erratically absorbed from the site, besides being very painful."

390. **The correct answer is (A).**

The answer is found in lines **1–3** of the paragraph: "In open-angle glaucoma a physical blockage occurs within the trabecular meshwork that retards elimination.

391. **The correct answer is (C).**

The answer is found in lines **8–9** of the paragraph. The normal intraocular pressure is 10-20 mmHg.

392. **The correct answer is (C).**

The answer is found in lines **10–12** of the paragraph. Visual field effects occur eventually and only after the disease has been present for a period of time. The changes are not immediate.

393. **The correct answer is (B).**

The answer is found in lines **6–8** of the paragraph: "The impairment of aqueous drainage elevates the intraocular pressure (IOP) to 25-35 mmHg."

394. **The correct answer is (B).**

The answer is found in lines **3–5** of the paragraph: "The obstruction is presumed to be located between the trabecular sheet and the episcleral veins."

395. **The correct answer is (D).**

The answer is found in lines **2–4** of the paragraph: "Besides loss of consciousness, these syncopal attacks involve pallor, muscular twitching, and sometimes seizures."

396. **The correct answer is (B).**

The answer is found in lines **18–21** of the paragraph: "An adverse dose-related effect is hypotension, which may occur by alpha-adrenergic receptor blockade or by a direct negative inotropic effect on the heart."

397. **The correct answer is (B).**

The answer is found in lines **4–6** of the paragraph: "When an EKG is obtained during an attack, the pattern indicates ventricular tachyarrhythmia."

398. **The correct answer is (C).**

The answer is found in line **1** of the paragraph: "An unusual reaction to quinidine is syncope."

399. **The correct answer is (C).**

The answer is found in lines **16–17** of the paragraph: graph: "Syncope may occur at low doses (e.g., 0.8 g/day)."

400. **The correct answer is (B).**

The answer is found in lines **1–3** of the paragraph: "Many reports have indicated that the tricyclic antidepressants, especially imipramine, may be of benefit in the treatment of MBD in children."

401. **The correct answer is (A).**

The answer is found in lines **10 and 11** of the paragraph: " . . . the maximum daily dose approved by the FDA (5 mg/kg per day) . . ."

402. **The correct answer is (C).**

The answer is found in lines **4–6** of the paragraph: "However, although most studies have indicated their superiority over placebos, they are still not as effective as the psychostimulants."

403. **The correct answer is (B).**

The answer is found in lines **15–17** of the paragraph: "In addition, the patient should be monitored for more severe effects on the central nervous system, for example, seizures."

404. **The correct answer is (D).**

The answer is found in lines **6–9** of the paragraph. "Further drawbacks associated with their use include the development of tolerance in some children and numerous deleterious side effects."

405. **The correct answer is (B).**

The answer is found in lines **8–10** of the paragraph: "Dextroamphetamine was initially used in 1937 and continued to be the agent of choice until the late 1960s."

406. **The correct answer is (A).**

The answer is found in lines **20–22** of the paragraph: "while proponents of dextroamphetamine indicate that, in their hands, it has comparable clinical efficacy at a lower cost."

407. **The correct answer is (D).**

The answer is found in lines **1–4** of the paragraph: "The primary agents in the treatment of MBD are the centrally acting sympathomimetics, for example, methylphenidate, dextroamphetamine, and magnesium pemoline."

408. **The correct answer is (C).**

The answer is found in lines **11–13** of the paragraph: "Methylphenidate usage increased in association with reports of a lower incidence of side effects with the latter drug."

409. **The correct answer is (B).**

The answer is found in lines **1–2** of the paragraph: "Procainarnide may be considered as an alternative to quinidine."

410. **The correct answer is (A).**

The answer is found in lines **12–15** of the paragraph: "Giardina et al. have intravenously administered 100 mg, up to a maximum of 1 g, every 5 minutes to treat ventricular arrhythmia."

411. **The correct answer is (D).**

The answer is found in lines **11–12** of the paragraph: "Procainamide may be given intravenously at a rate of 25–50 mg/min."

412. **The correct answer is (C).**

The answer is found in lines **3–4** of the paragraph: "Most patients absorb 75-95% of an oral dose."

413. **The correct answer is (A).**

The answer is found in lines **4–6** of the paragraph: "However, Koch-Weser estimated that 10% of subjects may absorb 50% or less."

414. **The correct answer is (B).**

   The answer is found in lines **14–16** of the paragraph: "The increase in intraocular pressure is approximately 10 mmHg for patients with preglaucomatous anterior chambers."

415. **The correct answer is (B).**

   The answer is found in lines **11–13** of the paragraph: "This ocular hypertensive effect is usually fully reversible within 1 month after discontinuation of steroid therapy."

416. **The correct answer is (B).**

   The answer is found in lines **17–19** of the paragraph: "In some cases, irreversible eye damage occurs if ocular tension persists for 1-2 months or longer."

417. **The correct answer is (C).**

   The answer is found in lines **2–4** of the paragraph: "This form of glaucoma is usually painless and involves no ocular findings or visual field defects."

418. **The correct answer is (B).**

   The answer is found in lines **22–25** of the paragraph. "Patients undergoing chronic topical steroid therapy should therefore have a tonometric examination every 2 months."

PART III

Pharmacy Education

ACCREDITATION OF PHARMACY EDUCATION

Pharmacy colleges are accredited by the American Council on Pharmaceutical Education (ACPE). The ACPE was established in 1932 and is the national accrediting agency in pharmacy that is recognized by the Secretary of Education, U.S. Department of Education, and the Council on Post-Secondary Accreditation (COPA). The ACPE is also a member of the Council of Specialized Accrediting Agencies.

The ACPE is an autonomous agency whose membership is derived through the American Association of Colleges of Pharmacy (AACP), the American Pharmaceutical Association (APhA), and the National Association of Boards of Pharmacy (NABP), with three members appointed by each of the respective associations. In addition, there is one member appointed from the American Council on Education (ACE). Thus, there are ten council members. Also, a panel of public representatives serves in an advisery capacity to the council and provides for public contribution to its proceedings. The American Foundation for Pharmaceutical Education provides major financial support for the council's general activities. The AACP, APhA, and NABP also provide annual support to sustain the council's activities.

A list of accredited degree programs published annually is available from the ACPE office upon request. Contact the **American Council on Pharmaceutical Education (ACPE),** One East Wacker Dr., Chicago, Illinois 60601; 312-664-3575; fax: 312-664-4652; www.acpe-accredit.org.

To be eligible to take the NABPLEX examination given by the respective states, students must graduate from a college or school of pharmacy that is accredited by the American Council on Pharmaceutical Education. Each state gives the examination with the exception of California, which gives its own examination. You should contact each state to determine when and how often the board examination is given and to ask any other specific questions concerning the requirements in that state. For more information, contact the **National Association of Boards of Pharmacy (NABP),** 700 Busse Highway, Park Ridge, Illinois 60068-2402; 847-698-6227; fax: 847-698-0124; e-mail: ceo@napb.net; www.napb.net.

INSTITUTIONS AND PROGRAMS

There are eighty-one U.S. colleges and schools of pharmacy as of this printing. Seventy-seven have accredited first professional degree programs, and four have programs in pre-candidate accreditation status. A few Pharm.D. programs have not yet been accredited by the ACPE. Contact the specific school of pharmacy for information on its accreditation status.

Twenty-six programs are in private institutions and fifty-five are in publicly supported universities. There are three independent, freestanding pharmacy schools, all private. The remaining seventy-eight schools are university affiliated. Thirty-five schools of pharmacy are part of an academic health-center campus.

Each college of pharmacy curriculum varies, but all have the same basic courses. The variation occurs in the course sequence, credit hours per courses, elective courses, and total number of hours required for graduation. Likewise, pre-pharmacy requirements will vary from school to school.

At the American Association of Colleges of Pharmacy (AACP) annual meeting in July 1992, pharmacy faculty members voted to move toward the Pharm.D. as the only entry-level professional degree in pharmacy. The American Council on Pharmaceutical Education (ACPE), in July of 1997, adopted new accreditation standards and guidelines that, when fully implemented, will result in only schools or colleges who offer the Pharm.D. degree being accredited.

PHARMACY STUDENTS

Pharmacy student enrollment ranged from 113 to 1,412 students per school in 1997–98. Schools report an application to enrollment ratio of approximately 3.1:1. The AACP's annual Applicant Pool Survey indicated that from September 1997 through August 1998, 25,161 applications were received by the seventy-nine schools of pharmacy reporting this data. There was a 10.5 percent increase from the previous year. According to the survey, women's applications represented 64.6 percent and men's 34.4 percent. Applications from African Americans represented 9.0 percent of the total for 1997–98; Hispanic applications, 3.6 percent; and Native American applications, 0.4 percent. Of the applicants in 1997–98, 35.3 percent had a previous degree: associate degree, 4.9 percent; baccalaureate, 29.6 percent; master's 0.8 percent; and doctorate, 0.2 percent.

The total full-time pharmacy professional student enrollment in first professional degree programs was 33,090 in the fall of 1998. Of these, 12,248 were enrolled in B.S. programs and 20,842 in Pharm.D. degree programs. Over 64 percent of the total students were women, and over 12 percent were minority students: African American (8.4 percent), Hispanic (3 percent), and Native American (less than 1 percent). Pharmacy school professional student enrollments peaked in 1975, having increased 56 percent since 1970. Enrollment declined steadily between 1975 and 1983; however, a 43 percent increase in enrollments occurred between 1984–85 and 1995–96. Attrition (tracking enrollees through to graduation) has decreased from a high of 15.5 percent in 1985 to 11.4 percent in 1998.

Total full-time graduate student enrollment in 1998 was 2,791: 2,088 students in Ph.D. and 783 in M.S. programs. 53.4 percent of full-time graduate students were men, and 46.6 percent were women.

The total number of professional degrees conferred in 1998 was 7,400, a decrease of 4.8 percent from 1996–97. Women received 64.2 percent of the first professional degrees, with men receiving 35.8 percent. Of the first professional degrees conferred, 64.4 percent were B.S. and 35.6 percent were Pharm.D. This was an increase of 17.3 percent in the number of Pharm.D. degrees awarded as the first professional degree. The total number of M.S. degrees conferred was 421 (an of 5.3 percent from 1996–97), and there were 411 Ph.D. degrees awarded (an increase of 14.8 percent).

*Data from the AACP Profile of Students Report, August, 1999.

DEGREE CHOICES

As a prospective pharmacy student, what choice should you make in selecting your pharmacy degree program? Should you enter a B.S. or a Pharm.D. program? The ACPE has indicated that only the Pharm.D. degree will be accredited in the future (2004). Since the trend is for an increasing number of schools to offer the Pharm.D. as an entry-level degree or as the only entry-level degree, it seems unwise to seek a B.S. in pharmacy. Many job ads indicate Pharm.D. only. There are still jobs for the B.S. pharmacist, but as more and more schools offer the Pharm.D. and changes continue in health care, it would seem prudent to seek a Pharm.D. instead of a B.S. Please note that there are many competent pharmacists who hold the B.S. degree, and they are doing very well in the profession. However, for the future, the Pharm.D. is the degree that you should seek.

COMPONENTS OF PHARMACY EDUCATION

Pharmacy education can be divided into five distinct components:

1. **Pre-pharmacy education,** which requires two years as a minimum and may be taken at a junior college, community college, four-year college, or a university (time may be reduced by taking an accelerated load, although this is not necessarily recommended). Note that approximately 24 percent of students entering pharmacy in 1999 held a B.S. degree, and many students had three years of pre-pharmacy.

2. **Professional Pharmacy education,** which takes either three years (B.S. degree) or four years (Pharm.D. degree) and must be taken at one of the eighty-one accredited schools or colleges of pharmacy in the U.S. in order to take the NABPLEX examination for licensure.

3. **Graduate education,** which is comprised of graduate education that leads to a M.S. or Ph.D. degree.

4. **Residency or fellowship programs** following either the B.S. or Pharm.D. entry-level degree. These are one- or two-year professional experiences, which are offered in a variety of practice settings.

5. **Professional continuing pharmaceutical education,** which is a requirement for continued licensure as a pharmacist. Each state board of pharmacy has requirements for continuing education that is state specific. The majority of states require pharmacists obtain 15 contact hours (1.5 C.E.U.) each year to maintain their licenses.

DEGREES OFFERED

There are two professional pharmacy degrees offered by schools and colleges of pharmacy as the entry-level degree:

1. The Bachelor of Science in Pharmacy—B.S. (*Note:* **will be phased out by 2004**)

2. The Doctor of Pharmacy—Pharm.D.

The graduate degrees offered in the pharmaceutical sciences include the following:

1. Master of Science—M.S.

2. Doctor of Philosophy—Ph.D.

Fifty-six pharmacy colleges have graduate programs. The graduate programs in the pharmaceutical sciences at the master's and doctoral level include the focus areas of medicinal chemistry, pharmaceutics, pharmacology, toxicology, pharmacokinetics, drug metabolism, molecular modeling, and nuclear pharmacy. This list is not all inclusive. Many colleges also offer the Ph.D. and master's degree in health science administration, pharmacoeconomics, and pharmacy administration.

There are fourteen colleges of pharmacy that offer a joint Pharm.D./Ph.D. program. In these programs, students take all of their electives in the graduate school and must have a previous B.S. degree in an area other than pharmacy or three years of pre-pharmacy with significant course work beyond the pre-pharmacy requirements to enter the program.

Another very popular combined graduate program is the joint B.S./M.B.A. or Pharm.D./M.B.A. As of this printing, these programs are offered by thirteen colleges of pharmacy in conjunction with a School of Business. Students with the joint degree are very attractive to the government, the pharmaceutical industry, and the chain drug industry.

For information on graduate education programs and on joint undergraduate professional and graduate degree programs, contact the school or college of pharmacy that you are considering. You should also inquire about how many graduates enter residencies or fellowships following graduation.

PRE-PHARMACY REQUIREMENTS

Most pharmacy schools or colleges require two years of pre-pharmacy for entrance into the professional curriculum. Some programs have a 0–6 (pre-pharmacy/professional) program while others have a 1–5, 2–4, or a 3–4 program. A two-year pre-pharmacy curriculum includes either 60 semester hours or 90 quarter hours, depending upon the particular program. The following minimum requirements for admission are for the University of Tennessee College of Pharmacy and are provided for guidance only. Requirements for colleges of pharmacy will vary; the major difference will be the number of required hours in physics, organic chemistry, and mathematics. Students should contact each institution to which they are applying for specific information about that institution's requirements.

Minimum requirements for admission to the University of Tennessee College of Pharmacy are as follows:

1. Completion of 66 semester hours with 50 semester hours of required pre-pharmacy courses and 16 semester hours of elective courses.

2. PCAT is required at UT. A composite scaled score of 190 is required; however, this score is not a competitive score.

3. A personal interview and three letters of reference are required.

4. A grade of C or above must be obtained in each required course.

Pre-pharmacy Curriculum
University of Tennessee College of Pharmacy

Course	Semester Hours
General Chemistry	8
Organic Chemistry	8
General Biology/Zoology	8
Physics	8
Microbiology	3
English Composition	6
Communications/Speech (Interpersonal skills, not drama or theater)	3
Statistics	3

Fundamentals of Calculus 3

Social Science Electives 6
   (Psychology, Sociology, Economics,
   Anthropology, Political Science)

Humanities Electives 6
   (Literature, Language, History,
   Philosophy)

General Electives 4
   TOTAL 66

NOTE: One year of American History (high school or college level) is required for graduation from the University of Tennessee.

For information on pre-pharmacy requirements, graduate education programs, joint undergraduate professional, and graduate degree programs, contact the college or school of pharmacy that you are considering to determine the programs and requirements of that school.

PROFESSIONAL PHARMACY CURRICULUM

The professional curriculum in colleges of pharmacy has changed dramatically over the past twenty years. Until 1948, colleges of pharmacy required four years total education; however, today the requirement is five or six years, with two years to complete the pre-pharmacy requirements and three years in the professional curriculum for a B.S. and four years for a Pharm.D. Note that when the Pharm.D. is the only accredited entry-level degree, the total time required will be a minimum of six years.

The pharmacy curriculum is comprised of basic science and clinical science courses. The following are examples of two curricula, one a B.S. curriculum (generic program) and the other a Pharm.D. curriculum (The University of Tennessee). These two will provide you with an idea of the intensity and content of the pharmacy curriculum.

Bachelor of Science Curriculum (Sample Program)

First Professional Year	Clock-Hours per Week				Semester Hours	
	Lecture		Lab			
	semester		semester		semester	
Courses	1st	2nd	1st	2nd	1st	2nd
Medicinal Chemistry	3	2	0	3	3	3
Anatomy	3	0	3	0	4	0
Pharmaceutics	3	2	3	3	4	3
Pharmacology	3	3	3	3	4	4
Microbiology	0	3	0	3	0	4
Physiology	3	0	0	0	3	0
Health-Care Administration	0	3	0	0	0	3
TOTAL HOURS	**15**	**13**	**9**	**12**	**18**	**17**

MINIMUM CREDIT HOURS FIRST PROF. YEAR = 35 SEM. HOURS.

Second Professional Year	Clock-Hours per Week				Semester	
	Lecture		Lab		Hours	
	semester		semester		semester	
Courses	1st	2nd	1st	2nd	1st	2nd
Medicinal Chemistry	3	0	0	0	3	0
Biopharmaceutics	3	0	3	0	4	0
Therapeutics I	0	3	0	0	0	3
Introduction to Pharmacy Practice	3	0	3	0	4	0
Natural Products	0	3	0	3	0	4
Pharmacology	3	4	3	0	4	4
Pharmacy Law and Ethics	2	0	3	0	3	0
Electives	0	6	0	0	0	6
TOTAL HOURS	14	16	12	3	18	17

MINIMUM CREDIT HOURS SECOND PROF. YEAR = 35 SEM. HOURS.

Third Professional Year	Clock-Hours per Week				Semester	
	Lecture		Lab		Hours	
	semester		semester		semester	
Courses	1st	2nd	1st	2nd	1st	2nd
Pharmacokinetics	3	0	0	0	3	0
Therapeutics	4	4	0	0	4	4
Clinical Pharmacy Practice	0	0	20	20	6	6
Health Care Administration	0	2	0	0	0	2
Drug Information	2	0	3	0	3	0
Electives	2	6	0	0	2	6
TOTAL HOURS	11	12	23	20	18	18

MINIMUM CREDIT HOURS THIRD PROF. YEAR = 36 SEM. HOURS.

The bachelor of science in pharmacy is three professional years with a minimum of 400 hours (contact hours) of professional experience program and a total of approximately 92 semester hours of course credit during the three professional years. The following is a Pharm.D. curriculum that requires 152 semester hours for completion and has over 1,960 contact hours in the professional experience program.

DOCTOR OF PHARMACY CURRICULUM
(UNIVERSITY OF TENNESSEE)

First Professional Year

Fall Semester		Semester Hours	Lecture/ Laboratory
ANAT 111	Anatomy	3	(2/2)
BIOC 111	Biochemistry	5	(4/2)
PHSC 112	Medicinal Chemistry I	3	(3/0)
PPE 132	Intro. Pharmacy & the Health-Care Environment	3	(2/2)
PHSC 111	Physical Pharmacy	3	(3/0)
PHSC 113	Pharmacy Math	1	(1/0)
	TOTAL HOURS	18	(15 / 6)

Spring Semester			
PHSC 122	Medicinal Chemistry II	3	(3/0)
PHYS 121	Physiology	5	(4/1)
PHSC 123	Pharmaceutical Technology	5	(4/4)
MICR 211	Microbiology & Immunology	4	(3/2)
PPE 121	Basic Clinical & Communication Skills	2	(1/3)
	TOTAL HOURS	19	(15 / 10)

FIRST YEAR TOTAL SEMESTER HOURS = 37

Second Professional Year

Fall Semester		Semester Hours	Lecture/ Laboratory
PHAR 211	Pharmacology I	4	(3/2)
PHSC 212	Parenterals	2	(1/3)
PHSC 221	Biopharmaceutics	3	(3/0)
PPE 211	Professional Practice Management	2	(2/0)
PPE 224	Introductory Clerkship	1	(0/2)
	Elective(s)	4	(varies)
	TOTAL HOURS	16	(12 /4)

Spring Semester			
PHAR 221	Pharmacology II	4	(4/0)
PPE 221	Selfcare & Nonprescription Drugs	3	(3/0)
CLPH 311	Therapeutics I	4	(4/0)
PPE 222	Drug Information & Literature Evaluation	2	(1/2)
PHSC 233	Pharmacokinetics	3	(2/2)
CLPH 324/325	Community/Institutional Rotation (May)	4	(0/10)
	Elective(s)	2	(varies)
	TOTAL HOURS	22	(14 / 14)

SECOND YEAR TOTAL SEMESTER HOURS = 41

Third Professional Year

Fall Semester		Semester Hours	Lecture/ Laboratory
CLPH 312	Therapeutics II	4	(4/0)
CLPH 313	Therapeutics III	4	(4/0)
CLPH 314	Applied Therapeutics	2	(2/0)
CLPH 315	Applied Pharmacokinetics	3	(2/2)
PPE 213	Legal & Ethical Env. of Pharmacy	3	(3/0)
	Elective(s)	2	(varies)
	TOTAL HOURS	18	(16 / 2)

Spring Semester		Semester Hours	Lecture/ Laboratory
CLPH 321	Therapeutics IV	3	(3/0)
CLPH 322	Therapeutics V	3	(3/0)
PPE 223	Patient Assessment	2	(1/2)
CLPH 323	Applied Therapeutics II	2	(2/0)
PPE 324/325	Community/Institutional Rotation	4	(0/10)
	Therapeutic Selective	2	(2/0)
	TOTAL HOURS	16	(11/12)

THIRD YEAR TOTAL SEMESTER HOURS = 32

Fourth Professional Year

Fall Semester	Semester Hours	Lecture/ Laboratory
CLPH 411 Clinical Rotation I	4	(0/10)
CLPH 412 Clinical Rotation II	4	(0/10)
CLPH 413 Clinical Rotation III	4	(0/10)
CLPH 414 Clinical Rotation IV	4	(0/10)
CLPH 415 Clinical Rotation V	4	(0/10)
TOTAL HOURS	20	(0 / 50)

Spring Semester	Semester Hours	Lecture/ Laboratory
Rotation (selective)	4	(0/10)
Rotation (selective)	4	(0/10)
Rotation (selective)	4	(0/10)
Rotation (elective)	4	(0/10)
Rotation (elective)	4	(0/10)
TOTAL HOURS	20	(0 / 50)

FOURTH YEAR TOTAL SEMESTER HOURS = 40

As you will note from the above curricula, there is a significant amount of basic science course work, including biochemistry, anatomy, physiology, medical microbiology, as well as pharmaceutical chemistry and pharmacology. Other required courses may include nonprescription products, communication skills, toxicology, and drug literature evaluation.

The clinical science area of the curriculum deals with professional practice. The curriculum of the final professional year is heavily oriented toward pharmacy practice. Students participate in rotations (professional experience program), where they learn to apply what they know (basic and pharmaceutical sciences) in actual pharmacy practice. At rotation sites, students are educated by practicing pharmacists alongside medical, nursing, and other health-care students in a "health-care team approach."

Students can obtain rotation experience in such settings as community pharmacies, drug information centers, adult medical units, pediatric units, psychiatric units, ambulatory clinics, long-term care facilities, pharmaceutical manufacturing firms, and nuclear pharmacies. At these sites, students provide a variety of services to patients, including dispensing medications, educating patients about their drug therapy, conducting medication history interviews, and monitoring drug therapy. They also provide drug information to other health-care professionals and serve as consultants when decisions are made on drug therapy.

The Pharm.D. curricula require a minimum of 1,500 hours of professional practice experience. The University of Tennessee requires 1,960 hours of rotation experience. These hours are obtained by completing 12 one-month experiences of 160 hours per month. The above description is for a Pharm.D. curriculum. The amount of clinical experience required in a B.S. program is a minimum of 400 hours of rotation versus 1,500 hours in Pharm.D. programs.

Both degrees are considered entry-level degrees for the profession of pharmacy. The ACPE has recommended that all schools offer the Pharm.D. degree as the entry-level degree in pharmacy. For information on each pharmacy college's curriculum, you should write to the dean's office of the college in which you are interested. See the list of schools at the back of the book for contact information.

HEALTH PROFESSION ADVISERS

Pharmacy is an ever-changing profession, as are the educational programs of the pharmacy colleges. Most major colleges, as well as community colleges, have health profession advisers who can assist you in determining what courses apply to the pharmacy school of your choice as requirements for admission. Students currently enrolled in an institution that does not have a college of pharmacy should seek advice from their health professions adviser and particularly from the pre-pharmacy adviser. For more information on health advisers, contact the **National Association of Advisers for the Health Professions (NAAHP),** P.O. Box 1518, Champaign, Illinois 61824-1518; 217-355-0063; fax: 217-355-1287.

FREQUENTLY ASKED QUESTIONS ABOUT PHARMACY EDUCATION

How does the Doctor of Pharmacy curriculum differ from the Bachelor of Science curriculum?

The Doctor of Pharmacy (Pharm.D.) curriculum emphasizes a more patient-oriented course of study than does the B.S. curriculum. The Pharm.D. curriculum offers advanced courses in areas such as therapeutics, pathophysiology, biostatistics, and pharmacokinetics, which may not be required in the typical B.S. programs. It also provides an additional year of clinical (practice experience) clerkships/externships that are primarily devoted to patient assessment and counseling, drug therapy monitoring, as well as traditional dispensing roles.

Pharm.D. programs require a minimum of 1,500 hours of practice, while B.S. programs have a minimum of 400 hours.

Can students obtain a B.S. degree and then return for a Pharm.D. degree?

Yes, there are several schools that offer a post-baccalaureate Pharm.D. degree; however, their class size is very small, and admission is competitive. In addition, these programs are normally two calendar years long, which means it will take seven years to get the Pharm.D. degree rather than six years in an entry-level program.

What are the job opportunities for a Doctor of Pharmacy graduate?

Pharm.D.'s are qualified to do the jobs performed by B.S. graduates. Moreover, the Pharm.D. is qualified for highly specialized fields. (*Note:* At the 30th annual meeting of the American Society of Hospital Pharmacists, December 1995, over 60 percent of the jobs posted in the placement service showed preference to Pharm.D. graduates over B.S. graduates).

Can the Pharm.D. candidate specialize in a chosen area?

Most Pharm.D. programs have opportunities for students to take electives and to develop areas of emphasis such as the following: pharmacokinetics, metabolic support, nuclear pharmacy, pediatrics, drug information, mental health, geriatrics, infectious disease, home health care, community pharmacy, industrial pharmacy, and other specialty areas.

Are post-doctoral residencies available?

Upon completion of the Doctor of Pharmacy degree, there are a number of residency options available to graduates. The various programs include general hospital pharmacy residencies, specialty residencies, clinical residencies, and fellowships. A general residency or clinical residency is normally completed prior to the fellowship. Residencies are currently accredited by the American Society of Health-System Pharmacists (ASHP), and a number of new residency programs are being developed in community and other ambulatory care settings. Residency descriptions and information can be obtained from the American Society of Health-System Pharmacists. Residency programs in the community are detailed in information available from the American Pharmaceutical Association.

How will future roles of pharmacists differ from present roles?

The financing and organization of health care is changing rapidly. As the health-care system changes, so do the professions within the system. New laws in several states permit pharmacists to become actively involved in the prescribing of medications (called collaborative care agreements). We will see a continuous evolution of the pharmacist's role from being a dispenser of medications to that of a health practitioner with greater control over the selection, dispensing, and administration of medicines. Managed care and the market place are dictating major changes in the health-care system, and pharmacy is responding to those needs.

Do the anticipated changes in roles for the future necessitate a change in education?

Education will meet the future needs of the pharmacy practitioner. Greater emphasis is being placed on high technology, wellness-care, self-care, computer applications, and other innovations in order to prepare pharmacists for new responsibilities. Doctor of Pharmacy degree programs have evolved over the years in response to changing demands for specialized instruction and training. More pharmacists are continuing in postgraduate education after their B.S. or Pharm.D. degrees to prepare themselves for specialty areas of practice.

What factors should be considered in selecting a program for my professional pharmacy education?

Choosing a college or school of pharmacy is an extremely important and often difficult decision. Many factors should be evaluated, but the primary goal is to select the program that offers the highest quality of education and level of service. The institution's commitment to academic excellence and genuine concern for the student's needs are also important selection criteria. The location and setting are important factors; specifically, the types and varieties of clinical training facilities. The degree that is offered by the institution, B.S. or Pharm.D., is very important as well.

FINANCIAL AID FOR PHARMACY STUDENTS

There is a variety of financial aid available for students studying pharmacy programs. You may, for instance, be eligible for one or more of the following federal aid programs:

- Pell Grants—federal funding available for students on a needs basis
- College Work Study—federal and local funds available to pay salaries for students working on campus
- Supplemental Educational Opportunity Grants (SEOG)
- Health Professions Student Loans (HPSL)
- Health Education Assistance Loans (HEAL)
- Veterans Benefits
- National Direct Student Loan Programs
- Federal Family Education Loans

For more information about eligibility for these programs and how you can apply, write to the United States Department of Education or call the Federal Student Aid Information Center at 800-333-INFO.

In addition to federal programs, most schools and colleges of pharmacy offer need-based and/or merit scholarships to students. Each college or school also has its own financial aid program and may offer loans, grants, and scholarships. You should request financial aid information from each of the pharmacy programs to which you apply.

Many private foundations and organizations also have scholarship programs. Most libraries will have directories listing foundations and other private grants to individuals. Libraries will also carry reference volumes that describe in detail all forms and sources of financial aid for undergraduate, professional, and graduate study.

POSTGRADUATE EDUCATION: RESIDENCIES AND FELLOWSHIPS

In 1953, the American Society of Health-System Pharmacists (ASHP) began the accreditation of postgraduate training programs in hospital pharmacy. These programs were called hospital pharmacy residencies. During the past twenty years, the proliferation of residency programs has been dramatic. The ASHP is the accrediting body for hospital pharmacy residencies as well as specialty residencies. There are more than 183 accredited residency programs in the United States, as well as other nonaccredited fellowship, residency, and specialty residency programs. This number is growing every year.

PHARMACY RESIDENCIES*

What is a pharmacy residency?

A pharmacy residency is an organized, directed postgraduate learning experience in a defined area of pharmacy practice.

What types of pharmacy residencies are there?

The most common type is the residency in pharmacy practice, which is conducted in an institution under the preceptorship of the director of the pharmacy department. The objective of residency training in pharmacy practice is to develop competent practitioners who are able to provide a broad scope of pharmaceutical services (clinical services, informational services, drug distribution services, product formulation, quality control, supportive administrative services, etc.). Training typically involves structured rotations within the pharmacy department as well as other departments in the hospital, conferences, seminars, research projects, and related activities. Many residencies also provide for limited experience in pharmacies in other hospitals or other organized health-care settings.

A second type is the residency in a specialty pharmacy practice area that emphasizes the provision of pharmaceutical care in organized health-care settings to a wide variety of patients. Although most of the resident's training takes place in an institution, less emphasis is placed on the overall operation of a pharmacy department than in the residency in a pharmacy practice as described above. Most specialty residencies are available only to those who have completed the Pharm.D. degree. These specialty residencies include psychiatry, drug information, pharmacokinetics, cardiology, geriatrics, pediatrics, nutrition, critical care, etc.

* From the ASHP publication What is a Pharmacy Residency? Reprinted with permission of the American Society of Health-Systems Pharmacists.

What is meant by an "accredited" residency?

The accrediting body for the types of residencies described above is the American Society of Health-Systems Pharmacists. The society grants accreditation to institutions that meet certain standards of practice and that have demonstrated that they can provide a good training program. Accreditation of a pharmacy residency program by the society provides a certain assurance to prospective residents that the program has met these basic requirements and is therefore an acceptable site for postgraduate training in pharmacy practice.

How many hours are required to complete a pharmacy residency?

A minimum of 2,000 hours of training extending over a minimum of fifty weeks is required in an ASHP-accredited residency program; this is the equivalent of one normal work year. Some residency programs are offered only in conjunction with an advanced degree (M.S. or Ph.D.) in a college of pharmacy or graduate school. Such programs are commonly referred to as "affiliated" residencies and generally require two years for completion. Residents in some affiliated programs pursue the residency on a part-time basis so there will be adequate time for course work, thesis research, and the other degree requirements. Many affiliated programs, however, allow the residency to be taken either before or after the postgraduate academic course work. Other residency programs ("nonaffiliated" residencies) are offered independently of an advanced degree and typically require one year of full-time work for completion. An applicant who already holds an advanced degree would normally choose one of these programs if he or she is interested in pursuing residency training.

Do residents earn a salary?

All accredited residency programs provide the resident with a stipend, although the amount varies from program to program, depending on such factors as the number of actual residency training hours per year, the value of any fringe benefits provided, and geographic location (cost of living). The stipends are generally too inadequate to cover living costs for a resident having significant family support responsibilities. The average salary for residents in 1999–2000 was around $29,000 per year. Furthermore, a residency, whether affiliated or nonaffiliated, requires a full-time commitment on the part of the resident and usually does not permit supplementing income through part-time employment. For these reasons, applicants with family support obligations should have financial resources in addition to the residency stipend upon which they can rely during the residency training period.

Who should consider taking on accredited pharmacy residency?

Any pharmacist or pharmacy student whose career objectives center around institutional or clinical pharmacy practice should give serious consideration to residency training. Because of the concentrated nature of the training in a residency program, an individual may develop competence in a broader scope of pharmacy practice in a one- or two-year residency program than might be expected from several years as a staff pharmacist with a fixed assignment. Many positions-available listings in the ASHP Personnel Placement Service specify completion of an accredited residency as an employment prerequisite.

What are the requirements for admission to an accredited pharmacy residency?

An applicant must be a graduate of an ACPE-accredited college of pharmacy (or must have graduated prior to the beginning date of the residency) and should have demonstrated an interest in and aptitude for advanced training in pharmacy. Some residencies require that the applicant be licensed to practice before entering the program, although others will accept applicants who have some limited internship obligation remaining for completion of state board licensure requirements. In the case of an affiliated residency program, the applicant must satisfy the requirements of the college of pharmacy or graduate school for admission to the advanced degree program, in addition to the requirements established by the institution in which the residency is offered. Residents in ASHP-accredited programs should be members of the American Society of Health-Systems Pharmacists. Students with B.S. or Pharm.D. degrees who are applying for postgraduate residency and/or fellowship programs should write to the **American Society of Health-Systems Pharmacists Residency Matching Program,** 7272 Wisconsin Ave., Bethesda, Maryland 20814; 301-657-3000; fax: 301-652-8278; www.ashp.org. A list of accredited residencies may be obtained from the ASHP.

PART IV

Pharmacy Licensure

INTERN LICENSURE

Upon registration in a pharmacy college or school, students are eligible to become pharmacy interns. Some states require that interns be licensed; students should check with the Dean's office of their college or school concerning internship requirements in their state. All states require internship hours (hours of practical experience in pharmacy practice under the guidance of a pharmacy preceptor who is a licensed practitioner in the state in which the student is registered). The minimum number of required internship hours is 1,500. The majority of state boards of pharmacy require 1,500 hours; these hours may be obtained during the summer breaks between the professional years in the college of pharmacy or after graduation. Some state boards of pharmacy require that a minimum number of these hours be obtained after graduation. The current trend has moved away from this so that students may take the state board of pharmacy examination in order to become licensed upon graduation.

The boards of pharmacy give students credit for up to 400 hours of internship credit obtained during the clinical curriculum of a college or school of pharmacy. Some boards give more than the 400 hours; some recognize the clinical experience in the Pharm.D. program for the entire internship hour requirements. For specific information on how many hours of internship credit will be granted and on the specific areas of practice that will be allowed for internship credit, the state board in question should be contacted. A listing of state boards of pharmacy follows later in this section.

PHARMACY LICENSURE REQUIREMENT

After graduation, students must take a theoretical and practical examination administered by a state board of pharmacy. The National Association of Boards of Pharmacy's standardized NABPLEX exam is administered by all state boards of pharmacy, with the exception of California, which makes up its own licensure examination. The NABPLEX is administered several times a year. Each state board adheres to a standardized set of dates for giving the exam. These dates can be obtained from each individual state board of pharmacy office.

One of the most important functions of boards of pharmacy is to protect the public health and welfare. Each state board must set standards of competence for the practice of pharmacy. State laws require the assessment of the proficiency of each candidate in the knowledge, skills, and abilities necessary for the practice of pharmacy. State boards use the NABPLEX to make that assessment. A candidate for licensure who passes this examination to the satisfaction of the relevant state board is judged to have the required proficiency in that state and can also practice pharmacy in other licensing jurisdictions that offer reciprocity.

The licensing examination, which is oriented toward professional practice, is a qualifying evaluation rather than a competitive test. The NABPLEX Review Committee has established standards of knowledge, skills, and abilities they consider essential for the practice of pharmacy.

NABPLEX is used to assess these standards and is one determinant of a candidate's qualification for licensure. By its nature, the examination emphasizes that facts and information are meaningless without the ability to apply them in a practical situation. Furthermore, it highlights the skills and abilities that must be maintained throughout the candidate's professional career. As of 1997, the NABPLEX examination is given by computer in most states. Contact the state board of pharmacy in your state for further information.

RECIPROCITY BETWEEN STATES

Reciprocity is the process of transferring a license from one state to another. Most states recognize the test scores from other states, with some exceptions, such as California, which requires pharmacists to take its own board of pharmacy examination before becoming licensed. The usual requirement is that upon completing the state board of pharmacy requirements of a particular state, an individual must practice one year before being able to reciprocate his or her license from one state to another. However, many states participate in the score transfer program, which transfers the NABPLEX test scores to another state. Each state law is different.

In order to reciprocate to another state, individuals must fill out the appropriate forms, which can be obtained from the National Association of Boards of Pharmacy and from individual state board offices. Most state boards of pharmacy also require a law examination along with the reciprocation papers. (The examination is on the federal and state laws governing pharmacy practice.) Specific information on reciprocation among various states can be obtained from the **National Association of Boards of Pharmacy,** 700 Busse Highway, Park Ridge, Illinois 60068, 847-698-6227; fax: 847-698-0124; e-mail: ceo@nabp.net; www.nabp.net; or from individual state boards of pharmacy.

STATE BOARDS OF PHARMACY

Alabama Board of Pharmacy
1 Perimeter Park South, Suite 425 So.
Birmingham, Alabama 35243
205-967-0130
Fax: 205-967-1009
www.albop.com

Alaska Board of Pharmacy
P.O. Box 110806
Juneau, Alaska 99811-0806
907-465-2589
Fax: 907-465-2974
E-mail: debora_stovern@dced.state.ak.us
www.dced.state.ak.us/occ/ppha.htm

Arizona State Board of Pharmacy
4425 W. Olive, Suite 140
Glendale, Arizona 85302
623-463-ASBP
Fax: 623-934-0583
E-mail: info@azsbp.com
www.pharmacy.state.az.us

Arkansas State Board of Pharmacy
101 E. Capitol, Suite 218
Little Rock, Arkansas 72201
501-682-0190
Fax: 501-682-0195
www.state.ar.us/asbp/

California Board of Pharmacy
400 R St., Suite 4070
Sacramento, California 95814
916-445-5014
Fax: 916-327-6308
E-mail: rxcontactus@dca.ca.gov
www.pharmacy.ca.gov

Colorado State Board of Pharmacy
1560 Broadway, Suite 1310
Denver, Colorado 80202
303-894-7750
Fax: 303-894-7764
E-mail: pharmacy@dora.state.co.us
www.dora.state.co.us/pharmacy/

Connecticut Commission of Pharmacy, DCP
165 Capitol Ave.
Hartford, Connecticut 06106
860-713-6065
Fax: 860-713-7242
E-mail: michelle.sylvestre@po.state.ct.us
www.ctdrugcontrol.com/rxcommision.htm

Delaware State Board of Pharmacy
P.O. Box 637
Dover, Delaware 19901
302-739-4798

District of Columbia Board of Pharmacy
825 N. Capitol Street, NE, Room 2224
Washington, DC 20002
202-442-9200
Fax: 202-442-9431

Florida Board of Pharmacy
NorthWood Center
4052 Bald Cyress Way, Bin #C04
Tallahassee, Florida 32399-3254
850-414-2969
E-mail: bobbie_sawner@doh.state.fl.us
www.doh.state.fl.us/mqa/pharmacy/pshome.htm

Georgia State Board of Pharmacy
237 Coliseum Dr.
Macon, Georgia 31217-3858
478-207-1686
Fax: 478-207-1699
E-mail: rfthompson@sos.state.ga.us
www.sos.state.ga.us/ebd-pharmacy/

Hawaii State Board of Pharmacy
P.O. Box 3469
Honolulu, Hawaii 96801
808-586-2698

Idaho Board of Pharmacy
280 N. 8th St., Suite 204
P.O. Box 83720
Boise, Idaho 83720-0067
208-334-2356
www.state.id.us/bop

Illinois Board of Pharmacy
Illinois Department of Professional Regulation
320 W. Washington St., 3rd Floor
Springfield, Illinois 62786
217-785-8159
www.dpr.state.il.us

Indiana State Board of Pharmacy
Health Professions Bureau
402 W. Washington St., Room 041
Indianapolis, Indiana 46204-2739
317-232-1140
E-mail: kburch@hpb.state.in.us
www.ai.org/hpb/isbp/

Iowa State Board of Pharmacy Examiners
400 S.W. Eighth St., Suite E
Des Moines, Iowa 50309-4688
515-281-5944
Fax: 515-281-4629
www.state.ia.us/ibpe

Kansas State Board of Pharmacy
Landon State Office Building
900 Jackson, Room 513
Kansas City, Kansas 66612-1231
888-RXBOARD or 785-296-4056
Fax: 785-296-8420
www.ink.org/public/pharmacy/

Kentucky Board of Pharmacy
1024 Capital Center Dr., Suite 210
Frankfort, Kentucky 40601-8204
502-573-1580

Louisiana Board of Pharmacy
5615 Corporate Blvd., Suite 8E
Baton Rouge, Louisiana 70808-2537
225-925-6496
E-mail: labp@labp.com
www.labp.com

Maine Board of Pharmacy
Dept. of Professional & Financial Regulation
Office of Licensing & Registration
35 State House Station
Augusta, Maine 04333-0035
207-624-8689
Fax: 207-624-8637
E-mail: susan.a.greenlaw@state.me.us
www.state.me.us/pfr/led/pharmacy/index.htm

Maryland Board of Pharmacy
4201 Patterson Ave.
Baltimore, Maryland 21215-2299
410-764-4755
E-mail: md_pharmacy_board@yahoo.com

Massachusetts Board of Registration in Pharmacy
239 Causeway St., Suite 500
Boston, Massachusetts 02114
617-727-3074
Fax: 617-727-2197
E-mail: charles.r.young@state.ma.us
www.state.ma.us/reg/boards/ph

Michigan Board of Pharmacy
611 W. Ottawa, 1st Floor
P.O. Box 30670
Lansing, Michigan 48909-8170
517-373-9102
www.michigan.gov/cis

Minnesota State Board of Pharmacy
2829 University Ave. SE, Suite 530
Minneapolis, Minnesota 55414-3251
612-617-2201
Fax: 612-617-2212
E-mail: pharmacy.board@state.mn.us
www.phcybrd.state.mn.us

Mississippi Board of Pharmacy
P.O. Box 24507
Jackson, Mississippi 39225-4507
601-354-6750
Fax: 601-354-6071
E-mail: pwoodberry@mbp.state.ms.us
www.mbp.state.ms.us

Missouri Board of Pharmacy
P.O. Box 625
Jefferson City, Missouri 65102
573-751-0091
Fax: 573-526-3464
E-mail: pharmacy@mail.state.mo.us
www.ecodev.state.mo.us/pr/pharmacy/

Montana Board of Pharmacy
P.O. Box 200513
Helena, Montana 59620-0513
406-444-3737
Fax: 406-444-1667
www.com.state.mt.us/License/POL/pol_boards/
pha_board/board_page.htm

Nebraska Board of Examiners in Pharmacy
P.O. Box 94986
Lincoln, Nebraska 68509
402-471-2115
www.hhs.state.ne.us

Nevada State Board of Pharmacy
555 Double Eagle Court, Suite 1100
Reno, Nevada 89511-8991
800-364-2081 or 775-850-1440
Fax: 775-850-1444
E-mail: pharmacy@govmail.state.nv.us
www.state.nv.us/pharmacy/

State of New Hampshire Board of Pharmacy
57 Regional Drive
Concord, New Hampshire 03301-8518
603-271-2350
Fax: 603-271-2856
E-mail: nhpharmacy@nhsa.state.nh.us
www.state.nh.us/pharmacy/

New Jersey Board of Pharmacy
P.O. Box 45013
Newark, New Jersey 07101
201-504-6450
www.state.nj.us/lps/ca/brief/pharm.htm

New Mexico Board of Pharmacy
University Towers
1650 University Blvd. N.E., Suite 400B
Albuquerque, New Mexico 87102
800-565-9102 or 505-841-9102
Fax: 505-841-9113
E-mail: nmbop@nm-us.campuscwix.net
www.state.nm.us/pharmacy/

New York State Board of Pharmacy
Cultural Education Center, Room 3035
Albany, New York 12230
518-474-3848
E-mail: pharmbd@mail.nysed.gov.
www.nysed.gov/prof/pharm.htm

North Carolina Board of Pharmacy
P.O. Box 459
Carrboro, North Carolina 27510-0459
919-942-4454
Fax: 919-967-5757
www.ncbop.org

North Dakota State Board of Pharmacy
P.O. Box 1354
Bismarck, North Dakota 58502-1354
701-328-9535

Ohio State Board of Pharmacy
77 S. High St., 17th Floor
Columbus, Ohio 43266-0320
614-466-4143
Fax: 614-752-4836
E-mail: exec@bop.state.oh.us
www.state.oh.us/pharmacy/

Oklahoma State Board of Pharmacy
4545 N. Lincoln Blvd., Suite 112
Oklahoma City, Oklahoma 73105-3488
405-521-3815
Fax: 405-521-3758
E-mail: pharmacy@oklaosf.state.ok.us
www.state.ok.us/~pharmacy

Oregon Board of Pharmacy
State Office Building, Suite 425
800 N.E. Oregon St. #9
Portland, Oregon 97232
503-731-4032
Fax: 503-731-4067
E-mail: pharmacy.board@state.or.us
www.pharmacy.state.or.us

Pennsylvania State Board of Pharmacy
P.O. Box 2649
Harrisburg, Pennsylvania 17105-2649
717-783-7156
Fax: 717-787-7769
E-mail: pharmacy@pados.dos.state.pa.us
www.dos.state.pa.us/bpoa/phabd/mainpage.htm

Puerto Rico Board of Pharmacy
Div. of Examining Boards, Office of Regulations &
Certification of Health Professions, Dept. of Health
Call Box 10,200
Santurce, Puerto Rico 00908
809-725-8161

Rhode Island Board of Pharmacy
3 Capitol Hill, Room 205
Providence, Rhode Island 02908-5097
401-222-2837

South Carolina Board of Pharmacy
P.O. Box 11927
Columbia, South Carolina 29211-1927
803-896-4700
Fax: 803-896-4596
E-mail: funderbm@mail.llr.state.sc.us
www.llr.state.sc.us/bop.htm

South Dakota Board of Pharmacy
4305 S. Louise Ave., Suite 104
Sioux Falls, South Dakota 57106
605-362-2737
Fax: 605-362-2738
E-mail: dennis.jones@state.sd.us
www.state.sd.us/dcr/pharmacy/pharm-ho.htm

Tennessee Board of Pharmacy
500 James Robertson Parkway
Nashville, Tennessee 37243-1149
615-741-2718
Fax: 615-741-2722
E-mail: klynch@mail.state.tn.us
www.state.tn.us/commerce/pharmacy/

Texas State Board of Pharmacy
William P. Hooby Bldg, Tower 3, Suite 600
333 Guadalupe St., Box 21
Austin, Texas 78701-3942
512-305-8000
Fax: 512-305-8020
E-mail: kay.wilson@tsbp.state.tx.us
www.tsbp.state.tx.us

Utah State Board of Pharmacy
P.O. Box 146741
Salt Lake City, Utah 84114-6741
801-530-6767
www.commerce.state.ut.us/dopl/dopl1.htm

Vermont Board of Pharmacy
Secretary of State's Office
Office of Professional Regulation
26 Terrace St., Drawer 09
Montpelier, Vermont 05609-1106
802-828-2875
E-mail: cpreston@sec.state.vt.us
www.vtprofessionals.org/pharmacists

Virgin Islands Board of Pharmacy
Dept. of Health
Roy L. Schneider Hospital
48 Sugar Estate
St. Thomas, Virgin Islands 00802
340-774-0117

Virginia Board of Pharmacy
6606 W. Broad St., Suite 400
Richmond, Virginia 23230-1717
804-662-9911
E-mail: pharmbd@dhp.state.va.us
www.dhp.state.va.us/levelone/pharm.htm

Washington Board of Pharmacy
Dept. of Health
P.O. Box 47863
Olympia, Washington 98504-7863
360-753-6834
E-mail: don.williams@doh.wa.gov
www.dpj.wa.gov/pharmacy/

West Virginia Board of Pharmacy
232 Capitol St.
Charleston, West Virginia 25301
304-558-0558

Wisconsin Pharmacy Examining Board
Bureau of Health Professions
1400 E. Washington
P.O. Box 8935
Madison, Wisconsin 53708
608-266-2812
E-mail: dorl@drl.state.wi.us
www.state.wi.us/agencies/drl/

Wyoming State Board of Pharmacy
1720 S. Poplar St., Suite 4
Casper, Wyoming 82601
307-234-0294
Fax: 307-234-7226
E-mail: wypharmbd@wercs.com
http://pharmacyboard.state.wy.us/

REQUIREMENTS FOR RELICENSURE

Requirements for relicensure varies by state. However, most states require mandatory continuing education. As of August 2000, forty-nine of the fifty-two boards of pharmacy require continuing education for relicensure. These boards are the following:

Alabama	Louisiana	North Dakota
Alaska	Maine	Ohio
Arizona	Maryland	Oklahoma
Arkansas	Massachusetts	Oregon
California	Michigan	Pennsylvania
Connecticut	Minnesota	Puerto Rico
Delaware	Mississippi	Rhode Island
District of Columbia	Missouri	South Carolina
Florida	Montana	South Dakota
Georgia	Nebraska	Tennessee
Idaho	Nevada	Texas
Illinois	New Hampshire	Utah
Indiana	New Jersey	Vermont
Iowa	New Mexico	Virginia
Kansas	New York	Washington
Kentucky	North Carolina	West Virginia
		Wyoming

The number of hours of continuing education that are required range from a minimum of 10 contact hours per year up to 30 hours every two years. Continuing education credits are defined in the following manner: one continuing education unit (1.0 CEU) equals 10 contact hours of credit. Pharmacists are required to report the continuing education programs attended to their boards of pharmacy.

The ACPE approves providers of pharmacy continuing education. The provider approval program assures pharmacists of the quality of continuing education programs by evaluating the capability of the providers of activities. Its aims are the following:

1. Advance the quality of continuing education, thereby assisting in the advancement of the practice of pharmacy.

2. Establish criteria and characteristics of approved continuing pharmaceutical education programs.

3. Provide pharmacists with a dependable basis for selecting continuing education programs.

4. Provide a basis for uniform acceptance of continuing education credits among the states.

5. Provide feedback to providers about their offerings, encouraging periodic self-evaluation with a view toward continual improvement and strengthening of continuing education activities. A pamphlet describing the standards for assessing and approving continuing education programs, as well as a list of approved continuing education programs, can be obtained from the **American Council on Pharmaceutical Education (ACPE)**, One East Wacker Dr., Chicago, Illinois 60601.

Appendix: Pharmacy Programs

Albany College of Pharmacy of Union University
Contact: Ms.Jacqueline Harris
Senior Assistant to Director of Admissions
106 New Scotland Avenue
Albany, NY 12208-3425
Telephone: 518-445-7221
Fax: 518-445-7202

Auburn University
School of Pharmacy
Contact: Dr. John F. Pritchett
Dean of the Graduate School
Auburn University, AL 36849
Telephone: 334-844-4700
E-mail: hatchlb@mail.auburn.edu

Butler University
College of Pharmacy
Contact: Dr. Beverly Sandmann
Principal Graduate Adviser
4600 Sunset Avenue
Indianapolis, IN 46208-3485
Telephone: 317-940-9553
E-mail: bsandman@butler.edu

Campbell University
School of Pharmacy
Contact: Dr. Daniel W. Teat
Assistant Dean for Admissions
Buies Creek, NC 27506
Telephone: 910-893-1200, Ext. 1690
Fax: 910-893-1937
E-mail: pharmacy@camel.campbell.edu

Creighton University
School of Pharmacy and Allied Health Professions
Contact: John J. Flemming
Director of Admissions
2500 California Plaza
Omaha, NE 68178-0001
Telephone: 402-280-2662
Fax: 402-280-5739
E-mail: spahp_admin8@creighton.edu

Dalhousie University
College of Pharmacy
Contact: Ingrid Sketris
Graduate Coordinator
Halifax, NS B3H 3J5   CAN
Telephone: 902-494-3755
Fax: 902-494-1396

Drake University
College of Pharmacy and Health Sciences
Contact: Dr. Renae J. Chesnut
2507 University Avenue
Des Moines, IA 50311-4516

Duquesne University
School of Pharmacy
Contact: Dr. R. Pete Vanderveen
Dean
600 Forbes Avenue
Pittsburgh, PA 15282-0001
Telephone: 412-396-6380

Ferris State University
College of Pharmacy
Contact: Dr. Rodney A. Larson
Assistant Dean
901 South State Street
Big Rapids, MI 49307
Telephone: 231-591-3780
Fax: 231-591-3829
E-mail: larsonr@ferris.edu

Florida Agricultural and Mechanical University
College of Pharmacy and Pharmaceutical Sciences
Contact: Carlton Bailey
Director
Tallahassee, FL 32307-3200
Telephone: 850-599-3039
Fax: 850-599-3347

Howard University
College of Pharmacy, Nursing and Allied Health
Sciences
Contact: Dr. Cecile H. Edwards
Interim Dean
2400 Sixth Street, NW
Washington, DC 20059-0002

Idaho State University
College of Pharmacy
Contact: Dr. Barbara Wells
Dean
741 South 7th Avenue
Pocatello, ID 83209
Telephone: 208-282-2175

Long Island University, Brooklyn Campus
Arnold and Marie Schwartz College of Pharmacy
and Health Sciences
Contact: Bernard W. Sullivan
Associate Director of Admissions
One University Plaza
Brooklyn, NY 11201-8423
Telephone: 718-488-1011
Fax: 718-797-2399
E-mail: attend@liu.edu

Massachusetts College of Pharmacy and Health Sciences
Contact: Ms. Lovie Condrick
Coordinator of Graduate Admissions
179 Longwood Avenue
Boston, MA 02115-5896
Telephone: 617-732-2986
Fax: 617-732-2801
E-mail: admissions@mcp.edu

Medical University of South Carolina
College of Pharmacy
Contact: Ms. Susan Coates
Pharmacy Admission Specialist
171 Ashley Avenue
Charleston, SC 29425-0002
Telephone: 843-792-8722
Fax: 843-792-3764
E-mail: coatess@musc.edu

Memorial University of Newfoundland
School of Pharmacy
Contact: Dr. Hu Liu
Graduate Officer
Elizabeth Avenue
St. John's, NF A1C 5S7   CAN
Telephone: 709-777-6382
Fax: 709-777-7044
E-mail: hliu@mun.ca

Mercer University
Southern School of Pharmacy
Contact: Dr. James W. Bartling
Associate Dean for Student Affairs and Admissions
1400 Coleman Avenue
Macon, GA 31207-0003
Telephone: 678-547-6232
Fax: 678-547-6063
E-mail: bartling_jw@mercer.edu

Midwestern University, Downers Grove Campus
Chicago College of Pharmacy
Contact: Ms. Julie Rosenthal
555 31st Street
Downers Grove, IL 60515-1235
Fax: 630-971-6086
E-mail: mwuinfo@mwu.edu

Midwestern University, Glendale Campus
College of Pharmacy–Glendale
Contact: Mr. James Walter
19555 North 59th Avenue
Glendale, AZ 85308
E-mail: mwuinfo@mwu.edu

North Dakota State University
College of Pharmacy
Contact: Dr. William H. Shelver
Chair
University Station
Fargo, ND 58105
Telephone: 701-231-7661
Fax: 701-231-7781
E-mail: fortier@badlands.nodak.edu

Northeastern University
School of Pharmacy
360 Huntington Avenue
Boston, MA 02115-5096
Fax: 617-373-8780
E-mail: admissions@neu.edu

Nova Southeastern University
College of Pharmacy
Contact: Margaret Brown
Admissions Counselor
3301 College Avenue
Fort Lauderdale, FL 33314-7721
Telephone: 954-262-1111
Fax: 954-262-2282
E-mail: mbrown@nova.edu

Ohio Northern University
Raabe College of Pharmacy
Contact: Dr. Robert McCurdy
Assistant to the Dean and Director of
Pharmacy Student Services
525 South Main
Ada, OH 45810-1599
Telephone: 419-772-2278
Fax: 419-772-2720
E-mail: r-mccurdy@onu.edu

The Ohio State University
College of Pharmacy
Contact: Ms. Kathy I. Brooks
Graduate Program Coordinator
190 North Oval Mall
Columbus, OH 43210
Telephone: 614-292-6822
Fax: 614-292-2588
E-mail: gadmbrks@dendrite.pharmacy.ohio-state.edu

Oregon State University
College of Pharmacy
Corvallis, OR 97331
Fax: 541-737-3999

Palm Beach Atlantic College
School of Pharmacy
Contact: Mrs. Carolanne M. Brown
Director of Graduate Admissions
901 South Flagler Drive, P.O. Box 24708
West Palm Beach, FL 33416-4708
Telephone: 800-281-3466 (toll-free)
Fax: 561-803-2115
E-mail: grad@pbac.edu

Purdue University
School of Pharmacy and Pharmaceutical Sciences
Contact: Dr. G. M. Loudon
Associate Dean
West Lafayette, IN 47907
Telephone: 765-494-1362

Rutgers, The State University of New Jersey, New Brunswick
College of Pharmacy
Contact: Dr. Joseph Barone
Director
New Brunswick, NJ 08901-1281
Telephone: 732-445-5215, Ext. 418
Fax: 732-445-2533

Samford University
McWhorter School of Pharmacy
Contact: C. Bruce Foster
Assistant Dean for Student/Alumni Affairs
800 Lakeshore Drive
Birmingham, AL 35229-0002
Telephone: 205-726-2053
Fax: 205-726-2759
E-mail: cbfoster@samford.edu

Shenandoah University
School of Pharmacy
Contact: Mr. Michael Carpenter
Director of Admissions
1460 University Drive
Winchester, VA 22601-5195
Telephone: 540-665-4581
Fax: 540-665-4627
E-mail: admit@su.edu

South Dakota State University
College of Pharmacy
Contact: Dr. Chandradhar Dwivedi
Coordinator of Graduate Studies
P.O. Box 2201
Brookings, SD 57007
Telephone: 605-688-4247

Southwestern Oklahoma State University
School of Pharmacy
Contact: Ms. Susan Thiessen
Admissions Counselor
100 Campus Drive
Weatherford, OK 73096-3098
Telephone: 580-774-3190
Fax: 580-774-7020
E-mail: thiesss@swosu.edu

St. John's University
College of Pharmacy and Allied Health Professions
Contact: Mrs. Patricia G. Armstrong
Director, Office of Admission
8000 Utopia Parkway
Jamaica, NY 11439
Telephone: 718-990-2000
Fax: 718-990-2096
E-mail: admissions@stjohns.edu

St. Louis College of Pharmacy
Contact: Ms. Penny Myers Bryant
Director of Admissions/Registrar
4588 Parkview Place
St. Louis, MO 63110-1088
Telephone: 314-637-8700, Ext. 1067
Fax: 314-367-2784
E-mail: pbryant@stlcop.edu

Temple University
School of Pharmacy
Contact: Dr. Cherng-Ju Kim
Director of Graduate Studies and Research
1801 North Broad Street
Philadelphia, PA 19122-6096
Telephone: 215-707-8173
Fax: 215-707-3678
E-mail: ckim0006@astro.temple.edu

Texas Southern University
College of Pharmacy and Health Sciences
Contact: Dr. Barbara Hayes
Dean
3100 Cleburne
Houston, TX 77004-4584
Telephone: 713-313-7164
Fax: 713-313-1091

Université de Montréal
Faculty of Pharmacy
Contact: Huy Ong
Vice Dean
CP 6128, Succursale Centre-ville
Montréal, QC H3C 3J7   CAN
Telephone: 514-343-6467
Fax: 514-343-2102

Université Laval
Faculty of Pharmacy
Contact: Monique Richer
Director
Bureau du Secretaire General
Quebec, QC G1K 7P4   CAN
Telephone: 418-656-2131, Ext. 5639
Fax: 418-656-2305
E-mail: pha@pha.ulaval.ca

University at Buffalo, The State University of New York
School of Pharmacy and Pharmaceutical Sciences
Contact: Dr. Wayne K. Anderson
Dean
Capen Hall
Buffalo, NY 14260
Telephone: 716-645-2823
Fax: 716-645-3688

University of Alberta
Faculty of Pharmacy and Pharmaceutical Sciences
Contact: Dr. Edward E. Knaus
Director of Graduate Affairs
Edmonton, AB T6G 2E1   CAN
Telephone: 780-492-5993
Fax: 780-492-1217

The University of Arizona
College of Pharmacy
Contact: Dr. J. Lyle Bootman
Dean
Tucson, AZ 85721
Telephone: 520-626-1657

University of Arkansas for Medical Sciences
College of Pharmacy
Contact: Dr. Kim Light
4301 West Markham
Little Rock, AR 72205-7199
Telephone: 501-686-5557

The University of British Columbia
Program in Pharmacy
Contact: G. D. Bellward
Associate Dean
1874 East Mall
Vancouver, BC V6T 1Z1   CAN
Telephone: 604-822-2390
Fax: 604-822-3035
E-mail: celineg@interchange.ubc.ca

University of California, San Francisco
School of Pharmacy
Contact: James C. Betbeze Jr.
Admissions Coordinator
Parnassus Avenue
San Francisco, CA 94143
Telephone: 415-476-2732
Fax: 415-476-6805
E-mail: jcb@itsa.ucsf.edu

University of Cincinnati
College of Pharmacy
Contact: Marcie Sedam
Assistant to the Director
P.O. Box 210091
Cincinnati, OH 45221-0091
Telephone: 513-558-3784

University of Colorado Health Sciences Center
School of Pharmacy
Contact: Dr. Carol Balmer
Director
4200 East Ninth Avenue
Denver, CO 80262
Telephone: 303-315-7709

University of Connecticut
School of Pharmacy
Contact: Gerald Gianutsos
Chairperson
Storrs, CT 06269
Telephone: 860-486-4066

University of Florida
College of Pharmacy
Contact: Dr. William J. Millard
Executive Associate Dean
Gainesville, FL 32611
Telephone: 352-392-8626
Fax: 352-392-9187
E-mail: millard@cop.ufl.edu

University of Georgia
College of Pharmacy
Athens, GA 30602

University of Houston
College of Pharmacy
Contact: Shara Zatopek
Assistant Dean for Admissions
4800 Calhoun Road
Houston, TX 77204
Telephone: 713-743-1262

University of Illinois at Chicago
College of Pharmacy
601 South Morgan Street
Chicago, IL 60607-7128

The University of Iowa
College of Pharmacy
Contact: Gilbert S. Banker
Dean
Iowa City, IA 52242-1316
Telephone: 319-335-8794
Fax: 319-353-5594

University of Kansas
School of Pharmacy
Contact: Jack Fincham
Dean
Lawrence, KS 66045
Telephone: 785-864-3591

University of Kentucky
College of Pharmacy
Contact: Ms. Patti Rutledge
Staff Associate
Lexington, KY 40506-0032
Telephone: 859-257-5303
Fax: 859-257-7297

University of Manitoba
Faculty of Pharmacy
Contact: Dr. Dan Sitar
Chair, Graduate Committee
Winnipeg, MB R3T 2N2   CAN

University of Maryland
Graduate Programs in Pharmacy
520 West Lombard Street
Baltimore, MD 21201-1627

University of Michigan
College of Pharmacy
Contact: James W. Richards
Dean
Ann Arbor, MI 48109
Telephone: 734-764-7312
Fax: 734-763-2022

University of Minnesota, Twin Cities Campus
College of Pharmacy
Contact: Marilyn K. Speedie
Dean
100 Church Street, SE
Minneapolis, MN 55455-0213
Telephone: 612-624-1900
Fax: 612-624-2974

University of Mississippi
School of Pharmacy
Contact: Dr. Barbara G. Wells
Dean
University, MS 38677
Telephone: 662-915-7265
Fax: 662-915-5704
E-mail: pharmacy@olemiss.edu

University of Missouri–Kansas City
School of Pharmacy
Contact: Shelly M. Janasz
Manager, Student Services
5100 Rockhill Road
Kansas City, MO 64110-2499
Telephone: 816-235-1613
Fax: 816-235-5190
E-mail: sjanasz@cctr.umkc.edu

The University of Montana–Missoula
School of Pharmacy and Allied Health Sciences
Contact: Dr. Vernon R. Grund
Chair
Missoula, MT 59812-0002
Telephone: 406-243-4765
Fax: 406-243-5228
E-mail: grund@selway.umt.edu

University of Nebraska Medical Center
College of Pharmacy
Contact: Dr. Edward B. Roche
Associate Dean for Academic Affairs
Nebraska Medical Center
Omaha, NE 68198
Telephone: 402-559-4334
Fax: 402-559-5060
E-mail: eroche@unmc.edu

University of New Mexico
College of Pharmacy
Contact: Susan Quintana
Administrative Assistant to the Dean
Albuquerque, NM 87131-2039
Telephone: 505-272-3241
Fax: 505-272-6749
E-mail: susanq@unm.edu

The University of North Carolina at Chapel Hill
School of Pharmacy
Contact: Ms. Sherrie E. Settle
Director, Graduate Education
Chapel Hill, NC 27599
Telephone: 919-962-0013
Fax: 919-966-6919
E-mail: sherrie_settle@unc.edu

University of Oklahoma Health Sciences Center
College of Pharmacy
Contact: Parke Largent
Director of Student Services
P.O. Box 26901
Oklahoma City, OK 73190
Telephone: 405-271-6595

University of Pittsburgh
School of Pharmacy
Contact: Anna M. Stracci
Director of Student Affairs
4200 Fifth Avenue
Pittsburgh, PA 15260
Telephone: 412-648-8579
Fax: 412-648-1086

University of Puerto Rico, Medical Sciences Campus
School of Pharmacy
Contact: Miriam Vélez
Assistant Dean of Student Affairs
P.O. Box 365067
San Juan, PR 00936-5067
Telephone: 787-758-2525, Ext. 5407
Fax: 787-751-5680

University of Rhode Island
College of Pharmacy
Contact: Louis Luzzi
Dean
Kingston, RI 02881
Telephone: 401-874-2761

University of Saskatchewan
College of Pharmacy and Nutrition
Contact: D. Gorecki
Dean
105 Administration Place
Saskatoon, SK S7N 5A2   CAN
Telephone: 306-966-6328
Fax: 306-966-6377

University of South Carolina
College of Pharmacy
Contact: Dr. Joseph W. Kosh
Graduate Director
Columbia, SC 29208
Telephone: 803-777-2705
Fax: 803-777-8356
E-mail: wise@cop.sc.edu

University of Southern California
School of Pharmacy
Contact: Dr. Timothy M. Chan
Dean
University Park Campus
Los Angeles, CA 90089
Telephone: 323-442-1369

University of the Pacific
School of Pharmacy
Contact: Ms. Cyndi Porter
Outreach Officer
3601 Pacific Avenue
Stockton, CA 95211-0197
Telephone: 209-946-3957
Fax: 209-946-2410
E-mail: cporter@uop.edu

University of the Sciences in Philadelphia
Philadelphia College of Pharmacy
Contact: Andrea Bagden
Secretary
600 South 43rd Street
Philadelphia, PA 19104-4495
Telephone: 215-596-8492
Fax: 215-895-1185
E-mail: flex@usip.edu

The University of Tennessee Health Science Center
College of Pharmacy
Contact: Ida Mosby
Director of Admissions
800 Madison Avenue
Memphis, TN 38163-0002
Telephone: 901-448-5560
Fax: 901-448-7772
E-mail: lmosby@utmem.edu

The University of Texas at Austin
College of Pharmacy
Contact: Ms. Mickie Sheppard
Graduate Coordinator
Austin, TX 78712-1111
Telephone: 512-471-6590
E-mail: mickies@mail.utexas.edu

University of Toledo
College of Pharmacy
Contact: Mrs. Sharon Troutman
Graduate Coordinator
2801 West Bancroft
Toledo, OH 43606-3398
Telephone: 419-530-1910
E-mail: stroutm@utnet.utoledo.edu

University of Utah
College of Pharmacy
Contact: Dr. John W. Mauger
Dean
201 South University Street
Salt Lake City, UT 84112-1107
Telephone: 801-581-6731

University of Washington
School of Pharmacy
Contact: Dr. Sid Nelson
Dean
Seattle, WA 98195
Telephone: 206-543-2030
Fax: 206-685-9297
E-mail: pha@u.washington.edu

University of Wisconsin--Madison
School of Pharmacy
Contact: Ms. Linda R. Frei
Graduate Coordinator
500 Lincoln Drive
Madison, WI 53706-1380
Telephone: 608-262-1200
Fax: 608-262-3397
E-mail: lrfrei@pharmacy.wisc.edu

Virginia Commonwealth University
School of Pharmacy
Contact: Betty B. Dobbie
Assistant to Dean, Admissions
901 West Franklin Street
Richmond, VA 23284-9005
Telephone: 804-828-3001
Fax: 804-828-7436
E-mail: bbdobbie@vcu.edu

Washington State University
College of Pharmacy
Contact: Dr. William Faffett
Interim Dean
Pullman, WA 99164
Telephone: 509-335-4750

Wayne State University
College of Pharmacy and Allied Health Professions
Contact: Steve Siconolfi
Associate Dean
656 West Kirby Street
Detroit, MI 48202
Telephone: 313-577-5875
E-mail: sfs@wizard.pharm.wayne.edu

West Virginia University
School of Pharmacy
Contact: Dr. Patrick S. Callery
Assistant Dean for Research and Graduate Programs
University Avenue
Morgantown, WV 26506
Telephone: 304-293-1482
Fax: 304-293-5483
E-mail: pcallery@hsc.wvu.edu

Western University of Health Sciences
College of Pharmacy
Contact: Kathy E. Ford
Director of Admissions
309 E. Second Street, College Plaza
Pomona, CA 91766-1854
Telephone: 909-469-5542
Fax: 909-469-5570
E-mail: admissions@westernu.edu

Wilkes University
Nesbitt School of Pharmacy
Contact: Dr. Bernard Graham
Dean
170 South Franklin St, P.O. Box 111
Wilkes-Barre, PA 18766-0002
Telephone: 570-408-4280
Fax: 570-408-7828
E-mail: grahamb@wilkes.edu

Xavier University of Louisiana
College of Pharmacy
Contact: Cathy Jones
Admissions Counselor
1 Drexel Drive
New Orleans, LA 70125-1098
Telephone: 504-483-7427
Fax: 504-485-7930
E-mail: cjjones@xula.edu

Your everything education destination... the *all-new* Petersons.com

When education is the question, **Petersons.com** is the answer. Log on today and discover what the *all-new* Petersons.com can do for you. Find the ideal college or grad school, take an online practice admission test, or explore financial aid options—all from a name you know and trust, Peterson's.

www.petersons.com

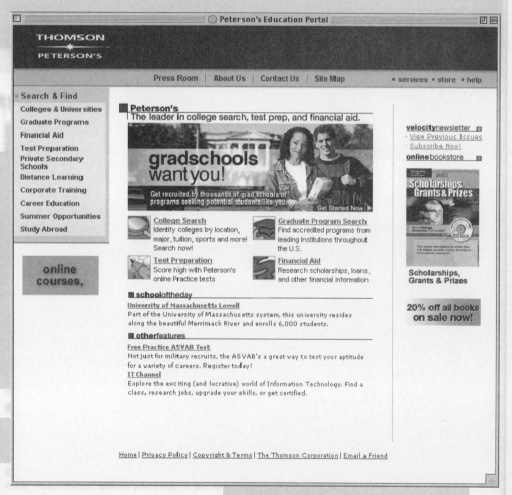

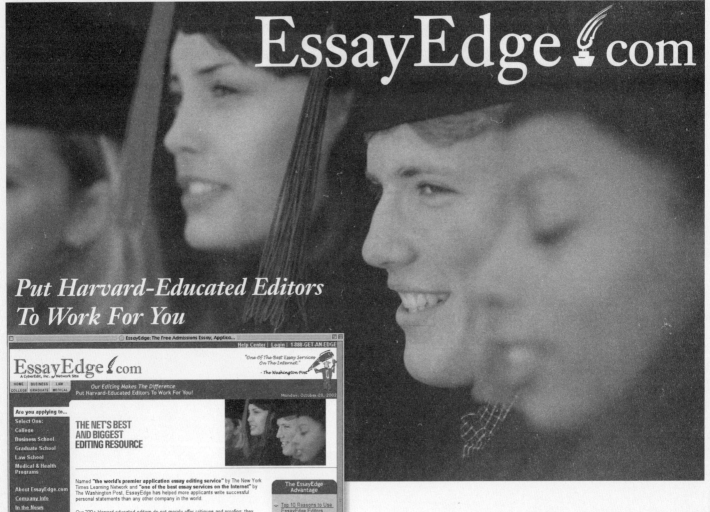
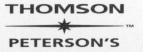